# Hair!

# GERSH KUNTZMAN

# HAIR!

## MANKIND'S HISTORIC QUEST
## TO END BALDNESS

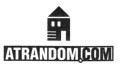

NEW YORK

Copyright © 2001 by Gersh Kuntzman

All rights reserved under International and Pan-American Copyright Conventions. Published in the United States by AtRandom.com Books, a division of Random House, Inc., New York, and simultaneously in Canada by Random House of Canada Limited, Toronto.

ATRANDOM.COM BOOKS and colophon are trademarks of Random House, Inc.

Library of Congress Cataloging-in-Publication Data
Kuntzman, Gersh.
Hair!: mankind's historic quest to end baldness / Gersh Kuntzman.
p.    cm.
ISBN 0-8129-9158-3 (pbk.)
1. Baldness—History.   I. Title.
RL155 .K86 2001
616.5'46—dc21    00-067540

Website address: www.atrandom.com

Printed in the United States of America on acid-free paper

2 4 6 8 9 7 5 3

First Edition

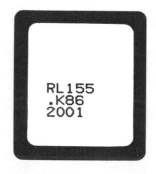

To Julie Rosenberg, the love of my life, and
to my parents, Ron and Bernice Kuntzman,
who gave me good genes—and
not only for hair.

# Contents

# Introduction

We are living in a golden age of baldness, my friends. Now, more than at any other time in human history, baldness is on the run—its cause understood, its treatment improved, its stigma vanishing.

Consider the advances in just the three major treatments for baldness, commonly referred to as "rugs, plugs and drugs":

• Rugs: Toupees—yes, there's that evil word—are better than they've ever been, thanks to advances in hairpiece technology and changing styles that were unthinkable a generation ago.

• Plugs: Hair transplants, once a crude operation involving the implantation of large plugs, can be almost undetectable today, thanks to single-hair grafts that mimic the scalp's natural growth patterns.

• Drugs: Medical science has not only figured out what causes baldness—a conversion of male sex hormones that shrink hair follicles until they die—but has also figured out how to prevent baldness from happening. There are two federally approved cures for baldness that actually work—Rogaine and Propecia—and more are on the way. The days of spreading hippo fat on a shiny pate (a Roman strategy), praying to the Sun god (Egyptian) or injecting candle wax under the scalp (a more recent, American idea) are over.

A golden age, indeed.

Yet the recent past is littered with the debris of failed promises, fake cures, misplaced hopes and bitter disappointment. Baldness—and the inability to cure it—took a profound toll on men, thanks, in part, to the social stigma associated with losing one's hair. While researching this book, I met bald men in doctors' offices as they awaited hair transplants, bald men in toupee salons as they tried to put a hairy bandage on their wounded pride, bald men in waiting rooms who just wanted to extend their Propecia prescription another six months.

But I also saw baldness from the other side, the men and women who are laboring—some would say heroically—to wipe out what one doctor once called "the scourge" of baldness and what one bald man once called "the most hideous, most loathsome, most detestable phenomenon that ever dawned upon mankind."

Just as a prior generation of doctors once obliterated smallpox, baldness is under attack from some of the most highly trained and gifted physicians and researchers of their age, people who could be curing cancer or AIDS but have chosen instead to battle a condition that affects more than 60 percent of men and 30 percent of women.*

Of course, there has always been some irony to male pattern baldness. It is caused, indirectly of course, by testosterone, the sex hormone that makes men men. Without testosterone, a man would have a high, squeaky voice, few muscles, weak bones, limited aggression and assertiveness, and little sex drive—in short, he would not be a man.

Yet it is the very sex hormone that makes us men that ultimately robs us of our manly mane. The result can be devastating (and not only because baldness tends to make us feel weak or impotent): A recent Harvard study showed that bald men are even more likely to suffer heart attacks and heart disease.

That decline of self-image and the desperation of bald men led directly to some of the horrors of the past—the snake-oil cures, the bad surgeries, the disgraceful prosthetics, a world in which every so-called medical practitioner was a charlatan (except for the one guy letting you in on the secret that everyone else was a charlatan).

---

*Another cause of baldness, the autoimmune dysfunction known as alopecia areata, attacks roughly one percent of the population. It is not addressed in this book, although its victims suffer the same loss of self-image and face the same challenges for finding a solution.

Vulnerable bald men have been preyed upon by shysters, sociopaths and ignoramuses—whose ilk is still with us today.

Yet times are changing. Baldness is becoming more and more socially acceptable. Maybe it started with Eisenhower ("I Like Ike"), our last—but hopefully not *the* last—bald president. Or perhaps it was Michael Jordan ("Be Like Mike"). But today, baldness is even considered fashionable.

One moment from history shows how far we have come.

In 1972, Wisconsin senator William Proxmire had the first of several hair transplant operations. A decade later, when he opposed New York City's proposal to build a new West Side expressway, then Governor Hugh Carey blasted Proxmire by telling the media, "I don't see how someone who had a hair transplant could be against a city having a face-lift."

Consider the outrage if an elected official said such a thing today, openly mocking an opponent's personal hygiene choices.

No less a barometer of the new chic of baldness comes from the late, great sitcom *Seinfeld*. Granted, the character George Costanza was agonized by his baldness and frequently used it as an explanation for his myriad failures in life. He even tried a toupee, with disastrous results (both for him and, subsequently, for toupee makers nationwide).

But it's telling that the one time he succeeded—he got a great job, he moved out of his parents' house, he dated an attractive woman— was when he embraced his baldness (inner and otherwise).

"Hi, my name is George," he told a woman at his favorite diner. "I'm bald, I have no job and I live with my parents."

She found him irresistible.

*Hair!*

# Chapter 1

—

# "A CURIOUS KIND OF PREJUDICE":

# THE PSYCHOLOGY OF BALDNESS

"Although the constitution makes no mention of it, it would appear
that fat people are now effectively excluded from running for high
political office. Probably bald people as well."
—NEIL POSTMAN, 1985

On the wall of an examination room in the office of New York
hair transplantation surgeon Dr. Michael Reed, strewn among
his diplomas, medical society membership plaques and a certificate
from a successfully completed liposuction workshop, is a framed
passage from the Bible.

Seeing two verses from chapter two of the second Book of Kings
on the wall of a cosmetic surgeon is somewhat startling—until it's
put in proper context.

In the chapter, God tells the prophet Elijah that He (God) is taking him (Elijah) up to heaven. Hearing the news, the great prophet
picks his friend Elisha as his successor (no doubt because the simi-
larity in names would avoid confusion among the masses), and the
two embark on a valedictory tour through Gilgal and Jericho. At the
border with Jordan, Elijah parts the waters and the two continue on.

Neither man, the record states clearly, discusses his hair in any
manner, although Elisha was, as we will find out later, bald.

After Elijah and Elisha arrive in Jordan, God sends a chariot of
fire drawn by horses of fire to deliver his faithful prophet to heaven

in a whirlwind, leaving the baldheaded Elisha to plot his next move. He quickly parts the waters and walks back to Jericho, a hardly subtle way of saying "I'm the man now."

"The spirit of Elijah," the Bible tells us, "doth rest on Elisha." Yet he was, the record states clearly, still bald.

Anyone who could part the waters and be fully accepted by his people as Elijah's successor (despite the total lack of democracy in the selection process) should have other things on his mind than his balding pate. But Elisha was a man like any other man.

And this is hair loss we're talking about.

After tarrying a bit in Jericho and miraculously replenishing the town's barren soil (he really *was* the Man), Elisha decides to leave the city, employing that classic show-biz strategy of leaving the people wanting more.

But on his way out of town, he runs into several children who mock him. Rather than turn the other cheek (hey, this is the *Old* Testament, remember), Elisha becomes consumed by his anger at being teased by the children.

And that is the subject of the framed passage on Reed's wall. In it, Elisha quickly violates the third and sixth commandments— Thou shalt not take the name of the Lord in vain, and Thou shalt not dispatch wild animals to tear apart a few wiseass kids:

> And as he was going up by the way, there came forth little children out of the city, and mocked him, and said unto him, "Go up, you bald head! Go up, you bald head!" And he turned back, and looked on them and cursed them in the name of the Lord. And two she-bears came out of the wood and mauled forty-two of them.

The biblical passage on Reed's office wall has a dual purpose. Of course it satirizes male vanity, but at the same time it also reassures Reed's bald patients that their obsession with hair is no mere symptom of today's orgiastic celebration of youth, but an ancient and still unresolved anxiety. While Reed's patients might choose a different method of retribution, they clearly see a small piece of themselves—successful, mature, adult men—standing on the roadside like Elisha, mocked for something completely outside of their control. Studies show, after all, that 60 percent of all bald men are teased at some point in their lives.

And, more important, the passage shows them that they are not alone: Baldness has been causing self-image problems for a long, long time.

In fact, the Bible, whose persistent refrain seems to be "Hair is good, bald is bad," plays a huge role in validating the prejudices of the nonbald [http://www.bible.org].

Take the much-cited Samson and Delilah story, the most high-profile example of biblical hair-ism. It is more than just a parable about betrayal and a strong statement about male virility. In fact, it's practically a commercial for Propecia.

In the story, an angel of the Lord comes down to Manoah and tells him that his barren wife will soon bear him a son who will "deliver Israel out of the hand of the Philistines."

Not a bad deal, but there's only one catch: "No razor shall come on his head," lest the boy lose his powers.

Everything goes according to plan; Samson slays a thousand Philistines with the jawbone of an ass and prepares to slay more when he meets Delilah, a harlot working the backrooms of Gaza. He falls for her like the mighty walls of Jericho, but she's a Philistine double agent and tricks him into revealing the source of his power (wow, the Good Book really *is* a good book).

"If I be shaven, then my strength will go from me and I shall become weak, and be like any other man," Samson tells Delilah in a moment of affection (for which he had, no doubt, paid in advance).

The rest, as they say, is the history of bald prejudice. But the Bible is only the jumping-off point. History shows us that hair has always been a powerful tool of subjugation and humiliation.

Roman obsession with hair nearly equaled our own—and like today, baldness was considered a scourge. Caesar, appalled that his naked pate projected an image of frailty, concealed his own baldness by combing his remaining strands forward, the antecedent of the classic comb-over that torments us to this day. Roman historian Suetonius captured it best when he declared Caesar a "dandy" and described his gratuitous use of laurel wreaths to cover his head.

"Of all the honors voted him by the Senate and People, none pleased him so much as the privilege of wearing a laurel wreath on all occasions," the historian wrote. "He constantly took advantage of it."

Of course, there was no end to the list of Roman "cures" for the blight, including pomades made out of hippo fat, salves containing the urine of young foals and liniments of sulfur and tar.

The Roman obsession with hair gave first-century satirist Martial (think of him as Tom Wolfe in a toga) a lot of material with which to work. The Spanish-born poet, who is best known for his twelve-volume collection of witty and deeply cynical epigrams, offered a condemnation of a Roman nobleman's futile efforts to conceal his baldness with a comb-over that could've been written (minus the flowery prose) today:

> From the one side and the other, you gather up your scanty locks and you cover, Marius, the wide expanse of your shining bald scalp with the hair from both sides of your head. But blown about, they come back at the bidding of the wind and return to themselves and gird your bare poll with big curls on the side and on that . . . Will you please, in simpler fashion, confess yourself old, so as after all to appear as a bald person. Nothing is more un-sightly than a bald man covered with hair.

What Martial failed to take into account, of course, was what it felt like to be bald in a society that despised baldness. It was bad enough being a slave in those times, but if you were a *bald* slave (talk about a double whammy!), you were believed to be fit only to clean toilets, stables and street gutters. Prisoners, adulteresses and traitors were typically shaved to heighten their humiliation, a practice that the French revived for Nazi collaborators during World War II.

And history has shown us—whether among the Maccabees in the

Bible, the Visigoths in the fourth century or Native American cultures more recently—that there's no better way to humiliate your vanquished foe than to slice off his hair or even scalp as a trophy. (As a badge of courage, many Native American warriors purposely left the frontal forelock on an otherwise shaved head, the better to facilitate the scalping should they be defeated in battle.)

You can try to put a positive spin on it—as the military does by making the bald head a symbol of obedience or as monks do by making the tonsure a sign of servitude to God—but baldness has never looked good to the wider society at large.

Face it, monks don't get dates.

Lest you doubt the weight of history that is carried on the back of every bald man, dozens of recent studies confirm that women and men typically prejudge the hairless as weaker, less potent, less friendly, older and, in one study, less "good"—especially when it comes to the all-important first impression.

"Bald or balding men may be disadvantaged in initial interactions, which may affect their social experiences and quality of life," said Thomas Cash, a psychology professor at Old Dominion University, who has studied the psychological impact of baldness for years [http://www.body-images.com/main.html].

University of Pennsylvania dermatologist Albert Kligman goes further: "Consider the consequences for a young woman whose hair has thinned out substantially by the age of twenty-five years. Can anyone doubt that this may seriously hurt her chances for dates and mates, for jobs, for achieving self-confidence—and so on, endlessly? . . . Those who are less beautiful or even unattractive are disadvantaged in virtually all human interactions."

Defying the stereotype that men are supposed to be Stoics about personal appearance and leave such frivolity to the fairer sex, bald men will often describe in painful detail their lives without hair: the teasing, the bad job interviews, the declining self-image.

"Maybe it's just middle-aged male vanity," joked Stewart, a fifty-one-year-old salesman I met in the office of New Jersey transplant surgeon Robert Bernstein [http://www.800newhair.com]. Stewart relaxed comfortably in a dentist-style chair moments before Bernstein was to carve out a swath of his scalp, dissect the thin pelt into individual hair units and then transplant the hairs into one thousand holes punched into Stewart's balding areas.

"I just know that I don't feel as good about myself as I was feeling when I had a full head of hair," Stewart said.

For "Carl" (not his real name), the problem on the top of his head went much farther down his body.

"I just don't feel like a man without my hair," he said while awaiting an appointment to get his hairpiece serviced at Penthouse for Hair Recovery, a locker-room-style hair salon for men who need a toupee and a reassuring slap on the ol' keyster [http://www.penthousehair.com]. "When I went bald, I wasn't the man I used to be."

Naturally, academics have done countless studies to put such real emotions into hard-and-fast scientific jargon.

In a 1971 study, for example, people were asked to look at random sketches of men and then asked to rate each man based on their all-critical first impression. The bald men were rated as the most unkind, ugly, hard and "bad." Men with hair were seen as more handsome, virile and active. Men with hair were also deemed "good."

One of my favorite studies—an examination of the perceived link between a man's hairiness and the length of his penis—shows that the notion of bald men as impotent losers is not something invented by the George Costanza character on *Seinfeld*.

In J. S. Verinis's study—aptly named "The Hairiness and Large Penis Stereotypes"—thirty-six male and twenty-four female college students were shown slides of a hairy and hairless arm, a hairy and hairless chest, a large penis and a small penis and were asked to rate the slides in adjectival pairs such as "good/bad," "kind/cruel," "virile/impotent," "strong/weak," etc.

Across the board, the hairy arm, hairy chest and long penis were seen as more masculine, more virile and stronger.

Verinis's conclusion: "Both men and women subscribe to this hairiness myth." My conclusion: "Hair makes the man."

Such studies launched an entirely new field of psychotherapy (and, of course, a new *name* for the new field): the study of the so-called physical attractiveness phenomenon.

Thomas Cash has made a good living studying the phenomenon—and has thrown good grant money after bad to conclude that people tend to find bald people less attractive.

Cash's 1988 study, for example, asked three groups of people—young college students, slightly older Old Dominion staffers and aging faculty members—to look at slides of bald and haired men. No one in the study was told why he or she was looking at these particular pictures, but was asked to rate the person in each slide for qualities such as self-assertiveness, social attractiveness, intelligence, life success, personal likability, physical attractiveness and perceived age.

Guess what? "The bald or balding models were perceived more negatively on every dimension except intelligence," Cash wrote. The study confirmed "a generally deleterious social stereotype of balding. Hair loss produced social judgments of lower aesthetic appeal and fostered less favorable initial assumptions about what the men were really like. Therefore, their lives were assumed to be less happy and successful. Both men and women expected the balding men to be less personally likable than the nonbalding controls."

University of Michigan professor Daniel Moerman did his own version of the study in 1988 (what, was grant money *easy* to come by then?), asking college students to look at two drawings of the same man—one with hair and one without—and give their impressions.

"The data indicate the existence of a curious kind of prejudice in our society," Moerman wrote. Across the board, the students thought that the bald subject was more intelligent, but considered the man with hair to be more attractive, more agreeable and younger.

"An opinion as to whether a person is agreeable or intelligent cannot be truly formulized until after direct interaction with the person," Moerman stressed. "The respondents in this experiment, however, were willing to predict that people would be more or less so after simply looking at a drawing."

And what they predicted was that men with hair, to put it in terms that one would hear on a college campus, are hotties and men without hair are, sigh, stable.

Researchers call this the "What is beautiful is good" syndrome—and even though it's been ingrained in our collective psyche since prehistoric times (from the cave paintings to *Charlie's Angels*), academics never stop writing about it.

"Physical attractiveness serves as an informational cue to infer extensive information about a person," psychologist Gordon Patzer wrote a decade ago.

"Consistently in our society, persons of lower physical attractiveness are associated with negative or undesirable characteristics, whereas their counterparts are associated with positive characteristics. People will adamantly state that another person's physical attractiveness has no effect on them, their perceptions, or their behavior; however, controlled observations reveal that people drastically underestimate the influence physical attractiveness has on them."

When an academic talks of "controlled observations," he is, of course, finding a rationale for doing yet another study. And that's exactly what the world got in 1990, thanks to a report in the *Journal of Nonverbal Behavior,* "Hair Loss and Electability: The Bald Truth," which sought to test the findings of guys like Cash and Moerman in a more practical setting: politics.

Do bald men face a harder time getting elected? Does a man with a good head of hair—think Ronald Reagan in 1980—convey a greater sense of vibrancy? Can a bald man ever be elected president again? And, more important, are these even rhetorical questions?

Apparently not. Earlier research revealed that better-looking candidates won an average of three times as many votes as their less attractive competitors. A subsequent study featuring six fictitious candidates of various degrees of physical attractiveness found that the top vote-getters among men were the three most attractive men (although for women voters, the study said, "the link between attractiveness and electability was less straightforward").

So, obviously, what was needed was another study. The first part of the electability study was straightforward: Although they could've easily been sitting around campus drinking coffee with shapely teaching assistants, the authors spent hours poring over photographs of all of America's top elected officials—senators, congressmen and governors. To keep the study as consistent as possible, the researchers eliminated anyone except white "Anglo" men. (As you might imagine, out of a possible 585 officeholders, eliminating all the nonwhite boys still left 522 men.)

From that point, the study was sheer arithmetic: Of the 522 officeholders, 328 (or 62.8 percent) had full heads of hair. And of the 194 (or 37.2 percent) who were balding, only 31 (or 6 percent) were in a state of "advanced baldness."

"Clearly," the authors suggest, "significant hair loss is the exception rather than the rule among high-level officeholders in the U.S., and advanced hair loss is rare."

But just how rare? Again, the authors crunched the numbers and discovered that if the officeholders' ages were taken into account and compared with societal averages, only 249 (or 47.7 percent) should have been expected to display no significant hair loss (instead of the 328), while 273 (or a majority of 52.3 percent) should have been thinning or bald (instead of the 194).

And instead of only 31 fully bald men in office, there should have been 118 (or 22.6 percent) if our elected officials resembled society.

"The number of bald or balding governors and members of Congress falls significantly below what would be expected of a randomly selected group of Anglo men of the same ages," the study concludes. "There is a bias against bald and balding men in high-level elective office."

This is especially ironic when you consider that baldness is indirectly caused by the very thing that makes a male a man: testosterone. In fact, most of the traits we commonly associate with masculinity—strength, a deep voice, a propensity to hurl insults at the screen when watching sports on TV—are a result of the very same male hormones that cause your scalp to lose hair.

Granted, Michael Jordan has gone a long way toward helping society reconsider its opinion of the bald man—but it also can't be ignored that his trademark bald head is a result of meticulous shaving, which allows Jordan to project the notion that his lack of hair is by choice rather than a deficiency, a weakness for which he would otherwise be negatively judged.

Perhaps Jordan, who started losing his hair shortly after joining the NBA following college, knew that athletes whose hair is noticeably thinning lose the respect of their teammates and fans.

Or, as *New York Times* sportswriter Richard Sandomir put it in his 1990 book *Bald Like Me:* "When sportscasters spot a bald athlete, they react as if they'd found he had no penis."

But were the bald men in the "Hair Loss and Electability" study less electable because they were bald or were bald men weeded out from the election process long before Election Day? Such a question, at least when asked on a college campus, cries out for another study, which is what the same authors did.

The second part of their analysis got to the heart of the matter by asking 550 adults to review real-looking campaign literature for "Allen Jordan," a supposed candidate for Congress. The adults were told that the study was centering on "the ways political candidates present themselves to the public," and not, as it really was, a study of voters' knee-jerk prejudice against the unhaired.

And just who was "Allen Jordan"? That depended on which brochure you got. Six male models—all bald—ranging in age from twenty-six to sixty-six were photographed in their natural, hairless state and then with a good-looking, professionally made hairpiece. The before-and-after photos were identical—except for the hair.

Participants, who received only one of the twelve brochures, were asked to grade the candidate's competence, strength, friendliness, attractiveness, masculinity, intelligence, leadership ability, warmth, courage, femininity, forcefulness and kindness. They were also asked to indicate how likely they would be to vote for "Allen Jordan" on a scale of one to one hundred.

The only downside of the study was that "Allen Jordan" did not exist, which is too bad, because, if the campaign literature was to be believed, Allen Jordan was just the kind of candidate for whom all of America is crying out.

Bald or not, the brochure showed that "Allen Jordan" was a true man of the people, "fighting with integrity" for the special needs of the homeless, the state's natural resources, health care for the elderly, tough penalties for drunk drivers, antidrug measures and no tax increases. And consider Jordan's impeccable personal life: He was a graduate of the state university, a military vet (no wimpy National Guard service for him), a business leader and a volunteer, a father of two, and a member of the state economic development board, the church council, the county historical society, the March of Dimes, the state's academy and the Optimists Club. He was identified as someone with "integrity, vision and sound American principles" (principles that, apparently, did not include having enough time to spend with those two kids of his).

So how did the bald "Allen Jordans" do compared with the haired candidates? Unlike in other baldness studies, there were no statistically significant differences regarding physical attractiveness, masculinity, dynamism or likability between the two groups. And the bald models fared just as well as the haired models on chance of earning the participant's vote.

So there's no bias against balding men, right? Obviously, you're not an academic. Of *course* there's bias, the authors said, but it didn't show up in this study because this study did not look at first impressions. In other words, the more you *know* about a bald guy, the less you find him repulsive. But if he's just some bald schmuck on the street, well, he's still just some bald schmuck on the street.

That's probably not such an overstatement. Disturbed by all these studies concluding that there's a bias against the bald, three more academics published a paper in the *British Journal of Psychology* saying that prejudice against the bald is a chicken-and-egg thing.

And the chicken is the bald man himself.

The paper, "Does Fortune Favour the Bald? Psychological Correlates of Hair Loss in Males," claimed that if bias against the bald really does exist, it's due to the bald man's lack of confidence.

Blaming the victim, indeed.

"[Bald men] are disadvantaged by their own negative psychological responses and self-perceptions," the authors stated. Among bald men going to psychiatrists, they noted, "problems most often mentioned were low self-esteem and clinical depression."

If the bald men would just get over themselves, everything would be fine and guys like "Allen Jordan" could enjoy unbounded success.

This attitude is pervasive in England—or, at least, in the ivory tower of English academia.

Shortly after the arrival of Propecia, a prescription drug that arrests the loss of hair in most men, a British doctor, Julian Barth, wrote that he didn't think men should even bother taking the drug.

"Whether [Propecia] will change the national history of hair loss or whether it will be useful in the prevention of baldness is not known," he said, ignoring reams of evidence of Propecia's utility. "Until then, men should still be encouraged to come to terms with their hair loss."

In other words, your hair may be falling out, your mood darkening and your chances for success going down the drain, but the solution is just to lie there and think of England.

Not that the British academicians didn't sympathize with the bald. "Does Fortune Favour the Bald" quotes at length a twenty-three-year-old Briton who had just survived a suicide attempt initiated, apparently, because his hair had begun to thin. His simple words give voice to legions of bald men.

"I just felt incredibly ugly—a bit of a freak," the patient says. "It just seemed so unfair and I was desperately unhappy. . . . I felt I had nothing to look forward to. . . . I haven't had a girlfriend now for two years. . . . I have much less confidence than I used to have and I don't work out nearly as much. . . . In a way I'm looking forward to getting older [because] being bald won't be so bad then."

In what could only be seen as an effort to drum up business in their psychological practices, the authors concluded that bald men are trapped in a catch-22 of mental health: Society discriminates against them because they're bald, so they become depressed and neurotic, which makes them even *more* likely to be discriminated against. And all the while, their hair keeps falling out.

"Far from being a laughing matter, male hair loss is clearly associated with a marked decrease in psychological well-being," the study concluded.

Who was laughing? Certainly not the World Health Organization, which actually classified male pattern baldness as a disease in 1992. And certainly not bald men. In subsequent chapters, you'll read about the makers of toupees, the developers of various medications to treat baldness, and doctors who perform hair transplant operations—all of whom are on the front lines of what I call mankind's historic quest to end baldness. Talking to their clients, customers and patients, I have found that the majority of bald men are profoundly affected by their lack of hair.

Baldness is an affliction whose psychological costs spare no racial or socioeconomic group. When John D. Rockefeller, Sr., the billionaire Standard Oil baron, went totally bald as a result of alopecia areata, the hair loss was his own personal Exxon *Valdez:* According to Ron Chernow's biography, *Titan,* Rockefeller aged a generation overnight and was unrecognizable to friends. Suddenly, he felt himself "a hairless ogre, stripped of all youth, warmth and attractiveness."

Rockefeller's morale was so devastated that he withdrew from social engagements and started buying every "remedy" he could find—an act of desperation that probably won't surprise most bald men. His weekly medication schedule called for six days of phosphorous and sulfur on Sunday because a doctor told him it would restore his hair.

Rockefeller eventually turned to wigs and was pleased with their results. He regained his personality and spent his old age as a veritable social butterfly.

Rockefeller's desperation was anything but uncommon. Where

bald men once suffered in silence, today there are countless web-sites and support groups devoted to helping men deal with their anxiety.

The Internet does ease a few furrowed brows as men begin to see that they're all in this battle together, but the immediacy of the Web allows rumors to run around the world several times before the truth has a chance to put on its toupee. The result, of course, are a lot of false dreams, dashed hopes and conspiracy theories.

On the Internet, I read a report of a promising baldness drug called RU 58841, created by the French drug company Roussel-Uclaf (the same company that brought us the far-more-controversial abortion pill). Several baldness websites were positively apoplectic about the pill's potential and angered that Roussel-Uclaf, which is now part of Aventis Pharmaceuticals, had supposedly tested the drug yet was unable, or unwilling, to bring it to market [http://www .hairsite.com/disc177_toc.htm].

Substantive information was limited. Aventis had stopped talking about the drug a few years earlier (and, indeed, declined repeated invitations to talk about the drug for this book). So without solid facts, conspiracy theorists had flourished.

And it's not just on the Internet. Bald consumer activist Spencer David Kobren says he gets regular calls to his weekly radio show, "The Bald Truth," about not only RU 58841 but many other "promising" treatments that, for some reason or other, have not made it to the market [http://www.thebaldtruth.com].

It has encouraged a cottage industry of anger to develop. I got a taste of this firsthand in an exchange of e-mails I had with a man who goes only by the nom de screen Maneless. I had posted a message hoping that someone in the baldness community knew more about RU 58841 and received a response from Maneless, who balked at telling me very much (being a conspiracy theorist, he was, naturally, conspiratorial).

But what I found most telling was the way in which his fear and paranoia, as they seemed to me, escalated to the breaking point even in just the few minutes it took him to bang out his response. His anger and frustration may be understandable only to bald men who have seen "cure" after "cure" turn out to be so much snake oil, but I had only asked Maneless what he knew about RU 58841. I was not prepared for the rage that was so close to the surface of his response. But he certainly had a lot to say, most of it a frenzied combination of anger, frustration and bitterness. Simmer for several years and serve hot:

I know that the company knows the drug is safe. I also know that the company knows that hair loss causes major depression, and the company basically does not give a damn if bald people suffer. I also know that the company knows that there have been suicides (and I believe more than have been officially documented) and the company does not care about that, so that means that the company does not care if more people commit suicide over baldness. I also know that the drug company has been approached by other huge major drug companies that wanted to buy the drug so as to bring it to market, but the company that owns the rights to the drug doesn't want to waste any resources on the drug at all, which it would have to do even if it licensed out the drug, so they won't license it out to other drug companies either. . . . I also know that the company knows that there is a lot of illegal drug and alcohol abuse over hair loss. I also know that the company knows that bald guys/women are taking drugs off-label (Cyproterone acetate for example) without being monitored to treat their hair loss. These drugs can grow hair but they are very toxic, and without monitoring the risk of death increases. . . . Bald people get them from Mexico and Canada, and then they take them here in America without being monitored. I know that women are taking these drugs off-label w/o being monitored sometimes and if they get pregnant the fetus could suffer severe deformities. . . . These people [the drug companies] are dogs. They have made a conscious decision to cause millions of innocent people to suffer. . . . The company really is run by a bunch of dogs who do not care about the suffering of innocent people. Why don't you snitch these bastards off in the media?

Don't be tempted to think of guys like Maneless as exceptions. Every new "breakthrough" meets with the same wave of euphoria, the overflowing of hype and then the crashing reality that the drug or treatment that is being touted won't be available for several years, if then. The result is increasing cynicism and mounting paranoia.

When a team led by Columbia University genetic researcher Angela Christiano reported that it had located a gene for a specific type of baldness, Christiano found herself inundated with offers from bald men and women to submit their own genes for testing.

One supposedly balding woman in Hawaii even sends Christiano a bag of hair—dated and weighed—every month, hoping to provide the doctor with the material to speed her genetic research.

And last year, Christiano ensured that her phone would keep ringing by coauthoring a landmark British study that reported success in transplanting human prehair cells from one person to another—a huge development that could revolutionize the way in which hair is harvested.

"From the minute that report came out [in the journal *Nature*]," Christiano said, "people were calling me up begging to be in the 'clinical trials.' There are no clinical trials. That's years away."

Christiano has fully recovered from her own bout with alopecia areata—which, as opposed to the gradual symptoms of the far more widespread male pattern baldness, is an immune system failure that can suddenly leave people totally bald [http://www .alopeciaareata.com]. But her experience with alopecia areata, which affects roughly one percent of people, helps Christiano understand what is driving her bald callers.

"You can't trivialize what these people are going through," she says, pointing to the latest Ziploc bag of thick, black hair from Hawaii, which she keeps in an increasingly large pile by her desk, a reminder that all her work in the lab has a very palpable human dimension.

"Baldness overwhelms people."

## Chapter 2

—

# TESTOSTERONE: THE ROOT OF
# ALL EVIL, THE EVIL OF ALL ROOTS

"Fair tresses man's imperial race insnare
And beauty draws us with a single hair."
—ALEXANDER POPE (1688–1744),
English satirical poet

The only sure way to end male pattern baldness is castration. Sure, you could study your family tree all the way back to Java Man, but the only way to be perfectly certain that you'll grow a full head of hair is to get yourself castrated—surgically or medically—preferably before you enter puberty.

It made perfect sense to Hippocrates way back in 400 B.C. The great Greek medicine man—himself a legendary baldy—observed that eunuchs did not go bald. He never quite figured out why, but the mere fact that he studied the phenomenon earned him a place in the Pantheon of Baldness; even today, we call a classic case of baldness—an advanced case in which a man is left with only a ring of hair growing around the back of the scalp at ear level—calvities Hippocratica, or, in layman's terms, Hippocratic baldness.

Hippocrates was onto something, but not enough. Clearly there was something about eunuchs that rendered their bodies and faces hairless while their heads remained full of hair. Never quite figuring out the mystery, Hippocrates thought he could cure baldness with

opium and rose essence mixed into an ointment with wine, oil of un-
ripe olives or acacia juice.

For severe cases, he recommended a poultice of cumin, pigeon
excrement, horseradish and beet root.

This was not a cure.

Hippocrates' inability to solve the mystery is typical. In fact, history has been marked by a clear and complete lack of understanding
about the basic cause of male pattern baldness. The very word "alopecia," for example, is derived from the Greek word meaning "fox
mange"—coined in the mistaken belief that male pattern baldness
bore some causal relationship to spotty hair loss in elderly foxes and
dogs.

Before the Greeks named it, the ancient Egyptians were equally
curious about the causes of baldness. They even had doctors—
"physicians of the head"—who specialized solely in diseases of the
scalp. It is believed to be the first known medical specialty.

They specialized, but their work in wiping out baldness was, to
say the least, primitive.

One ancient papyrus refers to a "cure" for baldness that was
merely a paste consisting of "lion fat, hippopotamus fat, crocodile
fat, cat fat, serpent fat and goat fat" rubbed onto the bald scalp. Another papyrus contained a cure comprised of "toes of a dog, refuse
of dates and the hoof of an ass."

Despite a medical interest in baldness, Egyptians invented wigs
as a fashion statement rather than a way to hide hair loss.

The Egyptians also had a great suspicion about hair in general,
believing that it had great power. After each haircut, a person's cut-
tings were collected and disposed of properly, lest they fall into the
wrong hands and be used for evil.

Alexander the Great, who lived up to his superlative by hacking
out an empire that included modern-day Greece, Turkey, the Middle
East and Iran in 330 B.C., started the world on an entirely new path,
hairwise. Up to that point, many cultures believed that the hair
should be allowed to grow as the gods intended, with trimming done
only to facilitate eating or swinging a sword.

But Alexander became convinced that long hair and beards were making it easy for his enemies to decapitate his soldiers, thanks to the convenient handhold afforded by a long beard or a full head of hair. He ordered his entire army to be clean-shaven, a style that later caught on with the general public.

The new style only made the Romans even more obsessed with hair. Not only did Caesar cover up his own baldness with laurel leaves (Cleopatra sought unsuccessfully to cure her beloved's baldness with another useless Egyptian balm made of burnt domestic mice, horse teeth, bear grease and deer marrow), but Roman senators could be turned away from the legislature if they had not properly shaved, a manifestation of a culture that, like our own, put a great social price on appearance.

Then as now, baldness was considered a scourge (remember the bald slaves who were thought fit only to clean toilets, stables and street gutters?), so Roman "scientists," like their Egyptian forebears and their modern-day successors, concocted a variety of useless "cures."

Pliny, a Roman scholar and naturalist who lived in the first century, called alopecia "a disgrace" and believed it could be cured by anointing "the bald and naked places" with a "liniment with the roots of the nymphae and hemlock stamped together."

Pliny also liked the hair-restoring power of the "dung of mice" or the urine of an ass foal mixed with spikenard "to rectify the strong scent."

A century later, the Roman medical authority Galen wrote that baldness was caused by eating mushrooms and toadstools.

Such misunderstanding of the cause and treatment of baldness continued for centuries. In the sixteenth century, Hieronymus Mercuria wrote that a "radical moisture" of the scalp caused the hair to fall out. Three hundred years later, after Napoleon's army froze to death following an ill-conceived offensive against Russia in 1812, his chief surgeon, Barron Larrey, reported back from the front that bald soldiers succumbed to the cold first. Though there was little evidence to support his finding, the notion took root that bald men were somehow weaker, and somewhat frailer, than men with hair.

By the nineteenth century, anyone who had a printing press was cranking out one misguided theory after another. At the time, many people believed, for example, that helmets or other headgear could cause baldness.

"We generally find hair at the back of the head," wrote Tom Robinson in his treatise "On Balding and Greyness" (1882). "May it not be because the back of the head is not so much covered by headgear as the fore part?"

No, Tom, it may not be.

Vair Clirehugh, a barber at the corner of Broadway and Fulton Street in New York, wrote in 1835 that the cause of baldness was that newly prevalent luxury known as hot water. The only cure for hair loss, Clirehugh decided, was cold showers. "They [cold showers] ought to be in as common use as a change of apparel," he wrote in his long-windedly titled "A Treatise on the Anatomy and Physiology of the Skin and Hair as Applied to the Causes, Treatment and Prevention of Baldness and Grey Hair; the Removal of Scurf, Dandruff, Etc."

More than a century later, water was still being blamed (and not just for scurf!). A former soldier named Daniel Alexander wrote a bizarre report in 1942 called "Finally, the Truth About Baldness and Its Relation to the Men in the Armed Forces."

The "truth" was that showers—like those taken by military men, who lacked "the benefits of the bathtub that was theirs when home"—caused, for lack of a better term, "hair erosion."

"After eight years of continuous thought and consideration, I have finally solved this problem," Alexander wrote. "The same water that has meandered its way through rock in France to form the famous Pont D'Arc; the same water that has carved, with its slow and forceful onrush, the enormous natural bridges in Southern Utah; the same water that has bored into existence with its cutting power, the natural bridge in Virginia; this force of water, when applied to the hair, with pressure, is in my opinion, the main reason for baldness as we know it."

Perhaps dismissing the fact that natural bridges formed only after millennia of constant "onrush" whereas a shower is just a few minutes long, Alexander marched on. "The daily shower acts as a 'shock' to the nerves which are disturbed to the walls of the hair follicles. . . . So every sailor, soldier and Marine is letting the steady stream of water from his daily shower slowly and forcefully carve out a sorrowful-looking bald spot on his head [and] his morale, his very fighting power, has been needlessly lowered."

Alexander, who obviously had some showering issues, recommended that the army issue a uniform, a rifle and a shower cap to every soldier.

Wrong again.

Lacking a smoking gun, many theorists of the age believed that hair loss, like venereal disease, was the result of bad morals or unclean living. H. P. Truefitt, in his 1863 book, *New Views on Baldness: Being a Treatise on the Hair and Skin,* said loss of hair was due to nervousness caused by "want of sleep, grief and excessive anger."

Wrong, of course. If that were true, all of New York City would be bald by now.

For the most part, theories on the cause of baldness tended to track prevalent social theories of the day. In his 1928 book, *The Story of Hair,* Charles Nessler, a manufacturer of women's salon equipment such as the permanent-wave machine, let the prejudices of the era color his judgment.

In fact, to him, baldness in white men (he didn't seem to recognize any other kind) was nothing less than a race war. Nessler speciously claimed that newer, lustier, highly fertile immigrants from southern and eastern Europe had lots of hair while the baldness he noticed on WASPs and other northern Europeans was an indication of their weakened libidos, fecundity and, frankly, personalities.

He also feared Jewish immigrants, whose hair growth—and, therefore, virility—exceeded that of non-Jews by "at least five percent." He saw them and other immigrants as "bearded conquerors from across the ocean," and Americans were destined for "race suicide" unless they could reproduce faster.

Wrong. Baldness affects all of those ethnic groups equally. Now, if he'd targeted his nativism on Asians, he might have had something; baldness is far less prevalent in Asian countries.

Despite all these theories, a consensus was finally emerging that baldness did have a genetic component. Too many scientists observing too many bald sons of too many bald fathers couldn't help but draw that conclusion.

"The man who would avoid baldness had better use greater care in the choice of his ancestors," researcher H. Rattner joked in 1941.

A 1916 study by researcher Dorothy Osborn set back mankind's understanding of baldness for decades. Osborn assumed that, like eye color, there was a single gene that controlled baldness—and that it was passed down on the mother's side. Only years later did scientists realize that Osborn's landmark study was flawed: She had thrown out results from nonbalding women, skewing her results in favor of a single gene passed down from the maternal grandparents.

This theory so dominated the public understanding of baldness for so long that many people today still believe they are safe from baldness if their mother or grandmothers had full heads of hair. They are not safe (unless, of course, they've been castrated).

In retrospect, Osborn's study should have been rooted out immediately. As we know today, common baldness cannot be the result of a single gene because all cases of baldness are subtly different. If baldness were controlled by the expression of a single gene—like an on/off switch—all bald men would be bald in exactly the same way at exactly the same time.

Plus, any illness that affects more than one person per thousand, geneticists tell us, cannot be controlled by a single gene.

Even as scientists were making great strides, others during the famed "snake-oil era" from the late 1800s to the early 1930s were still proposing their own causes of baldness.

A classic tome of the period was *The True Cause of Baldness* by Isidore Nagler in 1922—and it warrants a digression.

As vice president of the Amalgamated Ladies Garment Cutters Union, Nagler was a well-known figure who would later go on to be one of the organizers of the 1936 World Labor Athletic Carnival, which was held in New York to protest the Nazi-run Berlin Olympiad.

Isidore Nagler was sympathetic to the plight of his fellow baldies—perhaps a little *too* sympathetic. "Baldness is a problem not in the least inferior to any of the 'social problems' of the day," he wrote. "It is the most hideous, most loathsome, most detestable phenomenon that ever dawned upon mankind."

At the time of Nagler's writing, shysters—Nagler called them "reckless profiteers"—were exploiting the bald with their potions and "fake medicines" such as Forst's Original Bare-to-Hair or Lotta Lox plant juice.

Like many bald men who wanted to rid themselves of the scourge, Nagler admits that he "bought eagerly any new thing and none was of any use." He even tried a mixture of sulfur and salicylic acid applied to his scalp with Vaseline. It did not work.

Nagler had no use for the theory that genetics played a role in baldness: "It is the easiest thing in the world to shift the blame on our dear ancestors," he wrote, condemning "the presently much discussed theory of Heredity," capitalizing it as if to mock its self-importance.

So, Nagler did what any self-respecting, moral man of the Roaring Twenties would do: Blame masturbation!

Yes, masturbation, which mothers since the Roman Empire have been saying would grow hair on your palms, was actually the cause of baldness.

The root of all evil was "our own ignorance and abuse of nature's laws," Nagler wrote. "Upon this rock do I build my castle. All who read these lines will be in a position to preserve their hair forever."

Nagler was very passionate about his theory, saying that he was moved to publish his book out of a deep-seated responsibility to save people from his fate: "I feel like a soldier on the front who, noticing his commanding officer committing fatal errors in his duty, puts him aside and takes over the command himself, untrained as he is, and thus saves himself and his regiment from defeat and annihilation."

Nagler was no scientist, just a skilled observer of the human condition, he said. But even he knew the need for, how shall we put it, experimentation to prove his thesis. If not, why should anyone believe him? Embarrassed and ashamed by the bald pate that telegraphed his own experience with violating "nature's laws," Nagler admitted to practicing self-love in what remains the English language's least erotic confession of masturbation: "I underwent sufficient trials and experiment to sufficiently warrant for the justness and correctness of [the theory]."

Lest anyone think that Nagler was lying, he offered a fairly accurate description of the masturbatory process, saying that baldness stemmed from the fact that onanistic pleasure required both physical action (the masturbation itself) and mental stress (putting in your mind a picture of actual coitus so that the physical action can go forward).

"He [the masturbator] makes use of his mental powers to create an allegory of the presence of his mate when performing the abuse. . . . The extraordinary forceful concentration that we impose upon the mind when masturbating causes perhaps the central nervous system to react upon the cranium, thus causing the expansion and induration of the same."

This, Nagler submitted, was different from normal sex, which "requires the whole strain of every part of the body" rather than an overexertion of one part—in this case, the imagination. The masturbator, he claimed, "imposes a double task upon his nervous system. But how long will the body as a whole stand for such tremendous exploitation of its nerve?" How long, indeed!

Nagler concluded that the masturbatory process—with the nervous system overburdened by its "double task"—restricted blood to the scalp. He claimed that the first signs of baldness would occur within six months of the first self-love session.

"There's no truth to his theory at all," said Ron Trancik, a senior director of research at Pharmacia & Upjohn [http://www.pnu.com], the company that developed Rogaine in the 1970s. "Masturbation has been blamed for everything from hair on the hand to worsening acne. But it causes none of those things. I hadn't heard anyone tie it to baldness, but it doesn't affect that, either."

Nagler was just one of dozens of bald men with inquisitive minds all promulgating their own causes of the dread defoliation—none of them correct in the slightest way, but all of them convinced of their validity.

In the 1930s, the "Sleep Theory" came into vogue, aided by competing pamphlets by Thomas Redican and Charles Ferrante, neither of whom had any real expertise except, as Ferrante put it, "closely scrutinizing bald heads."

In his 1938 pamphlet, "Your Hair, Retain It and Achieve Maximum Regain," Redican theorized that modern man had caused his own baldness because he was, in essence, living more comfortably than his ancestors.

His method of curing baldness, therefore, called upon men to "approximate the conditions that our ancestors experienced through natural living and from which we are continually receding."

The prescription? Stop sleeping on a flat mattress. "Obtain two small blocks, preferably of wood, of size one by one by one-half to three-quarters inches thick," Redican wrote. "Place these blocks under each support at the foot of the bed. . . . Next, gently set the pillow aside on a chair or table. . . . When you are in bed, slide to the edge and allow your head and torso to hang over the edge of the bed . . . for about twenty to thirty seconds, during which time shake the head with the motions indicative of yes or no as are used in conversation."

Redican explained that this was no overnight cure. Employing an elaborate calculation, the author explained that a nineteen-year-old would need only 1,560 hours in the tilted bed to counteract all his years of flat-sleeping. A thirty-year-old would need 18,720 hours, or nine years. And a fifty-year-old bald man should pretty much give up; Redican said it would take twenty-four years of reclined sleeping to reverse the damage.

Redican sent a copy of his "findings" to the American Medical Association, which reacted with horror. "The plan to block up the base of the bed . . . seems somewhat unreasonable," an AMA investigator wrote in an internal memo. "He does not seem to be promoting any product whatsoever; it seems to be nothing more than a pet idea which has broken into print . . . another example of an unmedical mind attempting to apply itself to medical problems."

Charles Ferrante, who wasn't selling anything either, was received with the same skepticism. Ferrante theorized that women did not lose their hair (a fallacy in and of itself) because their long hairs tended to get "exercise" during the constant tossing and turning of sleep while men, whose shorter hairs never reached the pillow, did not.

"Nightly, the hair on the back and sides of the male's head receives rubbing from moving from side to side on the pillow," he wrote. "But the top hairs do not. From infancy, parents should allow their boys [sic] hair to grow long like the women and Indians."

It should come as no surprise that one of the few remaining copies of Ferrante's book is kept in the American Medical Association archive's historical frauds collection.

In addition to bizarre treatises, other would-be scientists wrote their own modern-day papyri—and all spoke of cures that were just as useless as smearing hippo fat on a bald head.

During this period, the laboratory at the American Medical Association was at its busiest, analyzing hundreds of samples sent in by concerned—or, rather, duped—customers. The "secret ingredients" of these snake-oil products were almost always revealed as inert.

H. T. Hair Tonic? "A slightly turbid green liquid having a strong peppermint odor and containing ash, sugar and benzoic acid."

Marine Hair Oil Restorer? "Saponifiable oil, sulfur, oil of tar, lanolin and possibly oil of sage and oil of bergamot."

Mr. Dowling's Hair Treatment? "Red pepper, kerosene and carbolic acid."

Georgia O. George's Hair-A-Gain? "Essentially a mixture of petroleum products resembling kerosene and mineral oil with lanolin, soap and tar or a tar-like substance." The Hair-A-Gain liquid shampoo was essentially a solution of ordinary soap in water.

Vreeland's Hairerbs? "Glycerine, water and a trace of sage oil."

The AMA was also asked about dozens of mechanical devices

that purported to grow hair—and again, the agency did what it could to dampen hopes of obviously cure-weary men.

In 1929, an Indianapolis company unveiled a massage contraption called "the Blud-Rub," which consisted of an examination table with a headpiece made of four discs, each covered with 256 "magic rubber fingers."

"No scalp, however tight and contracted, can resist their slow, but positive relaxing action," the company promotional material stated, promising to aid blood flow to the follicles.

With a myriad of products claiming to do just that, an investigator for *Consumers' Research* magazine wrote sarcastically, "It is surprising that there are any bald persons left in the world!" The American Medical Association responded, "Seriously, the thing is utter humbug."

In 1934, the Evans Company—the same shysters who created the Evans Vacuum Cap around the turn of the century—unveiled the Evans Electric Comb.

"European doctors explain this phenomena," the promotional material stated. "The electricity through the curved double rows of teeth is able to reach all weakened hair roots—literally pouring its life-giving energy over them."

*Literally.* Naturally, the AMA received a cache of letters from hopeful sufferers wondering if, this time, someone was actually onto something.

Not this time. "The so-called Evans Electric Comb is, in our opinion, 100 per cent quackery," the AMA wrote back. "The statement that 'the gentle electric current in the Evans Comb acts upon the hair as water upon parched plants' is 'hooey' to the nth degree."

Company owner Mrs. P. W. Bell didn't do a great job of defending herself, either: "If there was a fraud," she said in a subsequent fraud trial, "it was lack of knowledge on my part."

Two years later, a Cincinnati doctor with obviously good connections to the local press unveiled a machine he called the Xervac (pronounced "Ex-ervac"), which used vacuum pumps to massage the scalp. Product brochures claimed that "thousands now bald can have hair [thanks to] a gentle but very positive method of reaching the deep-lying circulatory system of the scalp."

The brochure even had photos of a man and a woman enjoying their massage; the man, in a smoking jacket, reading and the woman knitting while wearing the absurd-looking, fez-shaped, brushed-aluminum Xervac cylinder on their heads.

The machine was immediately hailed by the *Cincinnati Post* as an "almost entirely perfect process and machine to prevent and cure baldness. . . . If complete tests prove what the first 150 patients treated indicate—one hundred percent results—he will have accomplished what scientists have striven in vain to effect for centuries." (Usually, you can't *buy* that kind of coverage—unless, of course, you *do,* which inventor Andre Cueto apparently did.)

Then as today, the imprimatur of credibility that a genuine newspaper article afforded Dr. Cueto's invention was mammoth. *Time* magazine later followed with its own report, which was so unhesitatingly positive that it must have been written by Cueto himself.

"It exercises the capillaries of the scalp," *Time* said, obviously putting journalistic skepticism aside, "and brings revivifying blood to the follicles."

The reporters also seemed to forget history. Cueto's invention was nothing more than a new version of the Evans Vacuum Cap, a so-called "scientific method of growing hair" that was created in 1905 and also utilized vacuum pressure to "provide the exercise which makes the blood circulate in the scalp [and] feed the shrunken hair roots."

That was ancient history in the fast-moving culture of "modern" America.

But all the positive publicity put Cueto's invention under the microscope. Records show that dozens of doctors and readers of *Time* magazine immediately wrote to the AMA seeking counsel on the device. The association sent out a standard letter to all queries: "Every so often, something is brought out as a new method of growing hair. They have their day and after a time are replaced by another method which promises miraculous results for the bald. . . . Once hair follicles are destroyed, there is no method that can revive hair." But the Xervac flourished for at least a decade. A file at the AMA headquarters closes with a final letter in 1948 asking for an update on Cueto's miracle machine. The association's bureau of investigation wrote back that the Xervac "had some vogue around 1936. That it was not successful is obvious, as one no longer hears of the device." So where does that leave us? Back to the eunuchs.

All understanding of male baldness can be thought of as existing in the years B.H. and A.H., as in "Before Hamilton" and "After Hamilton." That's how monumental was anatomist James Hamilton's study "Male Hormone Stimulation Is Prerequisite and an Incitant in Common Baldness," first published by the *American Journal of Anatomy* in 1942.

Like Hippocrates, Hamilton was fascinated by castrati. But unlike in Hippocrates' time, when trustworthy eunuchs were created to guard harems, Hamilton's sample population consisted of men who were castrated by the criminal justice system, which in those days favored the procedure for violent sexual offenders.

"Jim was very interested in why people lost their hair," said New York dermatologist Norman Orentreich, who invented the modern hair transplant in 1952 by adapting some of Hamilton's research to the surgical arena. And, Orentreich said, there were plenty of castrati to study. "This was before the Nuremberg trials, so if a mentally defective male raped a woman, it was legal to castrate him."

Science, like everything else from the invention of the Toll House cookie to the telephone, sometimes depends on luck. One day, when Hamilton was examining a fully haired eunuch in a prison cell in Oklahoma, the man's identical twin brother—fully bald—came in for a visit.

It had long been concluded that genetics played a role in baldness, but standing right in front of Hamilton was the ultimate genetic question: How could two men, with the same genes, have such different heads of hair?

It had to be the testosterone.

Scouring the prisons of Oklahoma and other states, Hamilton rounded up a study group of 104 eunuchs—twenty men who had been castrated or otherwise lost the ability to produce testosterone before puberty, thirty-four during puberty and fifty after puberty.

A basic examination of the now grown men was telling: Of the fifty-four men who had become eunuchs before completing puberty, none was bald.

"Even the recession of the line of hair on the temples and the foreheads, which is observed in the majority of normal men, failed to appear," Hamilton wrote.

There it was, the secret to avoiding baldness: Go to the Castration Club for Men before you hit thirteen.

Sure, some of the thirty-four men from the "during puberty" group had begun to show the first signs of baldness—especially the guys who underwent the orchidectomy toward the end of puberty—but none had entered a state of noticeable hair loss.

In the final group, some of the fifty men castrated between ages twenty and forty-three had some hair loss, but the "loss of hair . . . occurred prior to orchidectomy." After castration, none had experienced further hair loss. At all.

But determining a connection between testosterone production and baldness was only part of Hamilton's genius. The biggest breakthrough came when Hamilton connected the genetic cause of baldness to the hormonal cause. After all, just as some children of bald men never go bald themselves, some of Hamilton's eunuchs would never have gone bald—even if they had not been castrated—thanks to good genes.

So Hamilton took twelve of the men who had been castrated as youngsters and injected them with testosterone. Four went bald almost immediately. Looking back into the family trees of these four men, Hamilton found that all came from families "in which normal adult male members tend to be bald."

He even stumbled upon one family of two eunuchoid brothers in which all but one of twenty-two adult male relatives in both maternal and paternal lines were bald. So when Hamilton started pumping testosterone into the two eunuchs' arms, they went bald, too.

And the eight other eunuchs who kept their hair despite the barrage of testosterone? They didn't go bald, Hamilton observed, because they "belonged to families without pronounced tendencies to baldness among the normal men."

This being a dry, scholarly paper, Hamilton was not in a position to write that he was, in fact, the Man when it came to discovering the causal relationship of genetics and hormones in baldness. Instead, he merely observed: "Concepts of the mode of inheritance in alopecia must be reformulated in view of the incitation of baldness by androgens. . . . A genetic tendency to baldness [is] dependent for fulfillment upon androgenic stimulation."

In his conclusion, Hamilton did allow himself one crack for the guys back in the lab: "Castration at early ages affords a reliable form of therapy, but one in which the cure is worse than the disease."

"He was a really remarkable man," said Orentreich. "In addition to being a great demographer, he was fascinated by all kinds of research. At the end of his life, he was working on a paper that the Scottish people were the lost tribe of Israel. He never really finished it."

When doctors today speak of Hamilton's work, it is not only with respect and admiration, but with a great deal of poetry. It is at such times, outsiders are reminded, that the creative side of science—the lyrical quality of a well-argued study or the artistic approach to the methodology of a particular research project—is often lost in the cold mathematical formulae and the rote injections of lab mice.

"Hamilton's work with the castrati was a beautiful example of observational clinical study," said Keith Kaufman, a researcher at Merck who helped develop Propecia a decade ago [http://www.merck.com]. "He not only noticed that if you didn't have testosterone, you didn't develop male pattern baldness, he noticed that the key factor was *when* you lost the ability to make testosterone. And then he closed the loop by observing his subjects when he gave them testosterone and analyzing their family trees. That was a beautiful series of experiments."

But as far as Hamilton took the science of baldness, he never quite figured out exactly how testosterone caused the hair on your head to fall out.

To understand that, it's first important to review the nature of hair biology (or, more accurately, the biology of hair nature). First of all, now that human beings have evolved to the point of wearing clothes and heavy winter coats, hair is something of a vestige. Less-evolved mammals rely on hair to keep them warm, whether by thickening in the colder months or just by holding in a layer of warm air close to their skins.

But we're so much more advanced than that. We wear fur. We no longer grow it for the winter.

Of course, there's another way of looking at it: "Hair is merely a useless load of stringy protein that's gotten excessively positive hype," wrote the famously bald *New York Times* sportswriter Richard Sandomir in his tribute to the hairless, *Bald Like Me.*

Hair itself is not living tissue, but a protein by-product grown in the base of the hair follicle by a rapidly dividing group of cells called the dermal papilla (think of it as a mini hair factory). The shaft of hair is pushed upward as a result of this rapid cell division at the base of the follicle. As the hair goes up the shaft, the living cells die and are keratinized—or hardened—as more cells grow beneath them.

Where does hair come from?

In the womb, hair germ cells, sometimes called hair peg cells, slowly sink from the primitive epidermis into the dermis during the early formation of the embryo while other cells are forming into the dermal papilla deeper inside the fetal skin. All this happens before the embryo is sixty days old. Both in utero and out, the dermal papilla is the most important part of hair anatomy. The signals it sends to other parts of the follicle—still not fully understood by modern science—affect every phase of the hair growth cycle.

The hair peg cells eventually differentiate into cells that form the different structures of the hair follicle, such as the sebaceous gland or the attachment site for the muscle that connects the hair follicle to the skin and causes the hair to stand up straight (as when you get goose bumps). The formation of those embryonic follicles is completed by the twenty-second week of pregnancy when lanugo hairs—fine, nonpigmented hairs—pop up all over the developing fetus's body.

The amniotic fluid is your first shampoo. But by the thirty-second to thirty-sixth weeks, all of the lanugo hairs on the scalp are shed into the amnion, to be replaced by normal hair (it's called terminal hair in scientific lingo); eyebrows and eyelashes also appear. Lanugo hairs stay in place over the rest of the body. Newborns finally shed it when they're three to four months old and begin growing terminal hairs.

By the time you're born, you've got all the follicles you'll ever need, all 100,000 to 150,000 or so of them on your scalp and 5,000,000 all over the rest of your body (except your soles and your palms).

Thankfully, unlike those of other mammals, all human follicles are not on the same growth cycle (if they were, you'd shed all your hairs at the same time and then have to wait a few months to get a new coat of hair). At any given time, 90 percent of your hairs are in the two-to-five-year anagen (or growing) phase and the remainder are in the two-to-three-month telogen phase (resting). Although science does not fully understand the chemical processes that trigger the switch-over from telogen to anagen and back to telogen, it is clear what happens biologically.

The anagen growing cycle begins to wind down when the dermal papilla cells stop stimulating growth. At this time, the hair follicle separates from the dermal papilla, sheds the hair and moves up the hair shaft—although like a breakup with a lover that doesn't "take" the first time, the follicle and the dermal papilla remain in contact. This process happens to everyone—even nonbald people lose 70 to 150 telogen hairs a day because they fall out during routine brushing or shampooing—but with bald people, those hair follicles will shrink and eventually die.

The chemical contact between the dermal papilla and the follicle is crucial, because a few weeks later, stimulation by the dermal papilla causes the hair follicle to descend and return to the anagen phase. As you can imagine, researchers are focusing a lot of attention on the signals sent by the dermal papilla, reasoning that if they can send them artificially, the hair follicle can remain in anagen permanently.

Like every cell in the body, the cells that rapidly divide to form the hair shaft are nourished with a constant flow of blood through tiny capillaries. This is perhaps why, decades and centuries ago, it was believed that poor scalp circulation was the cause of baldness. It is also why Orentreich was so easily able to transplant good hair into a barren area: The problem wasn't circulation in the bald area; the scalp is, after all, the most vascular area of the body. The problem was bad follicles.

Logic would say that this is impossible. After all, hair is evenly distributed over the rest of the body; you don't go bald, say, on one part of your arm while the other sprouts hair copiously. But the biochemistry of baldness turns even logic on its head.

The fact is, the crown and temple of a man's head—even those of a man with hair—are different from the back part of the head. Sure, it's all flesh and it's all properly vascular. The difference goes back to the womb. Even though we all start out as one cell, and then two cells and then four cells and then eight exact, same cells, eventually cell differentiation takes over as the body needs to start making muscle cells and nerve cells and brain cells and scalp cells. The problem is that a portion of the cells that are destined to be the top of your scalp (where you go bald) are derived from the embryo's neural crest, which itself comes from the ectoderm, while the back of your scalp (where you don't go bald) comes from mesodermal tissue.

Different parts of your head act differently. But to understand why follicles on the top of your head go bald and ones on the back don't, you have to go back to the poor, unfortunate eunuchs.

The primary difference between castrated men (especially those who were castrated before puberty) and intact men is that besides an inability to get dates, the castrated men have no testosterone, the principal male sex hormone (which earned its name from the testicles, where it is released).

At puberty, males begin producing testosterone, which causes muscles to gain strength, the bones to become more durable, hair to develop in embarrassing places, the voice to deepen, the genitals to enlarge, sperm to be produced, assertiveness and aggressiveness to increase and the famed male libido (long may it wave) to kick into high gear.

All that testosterone coursing through the teenager's veins means plenty of male hormones hitting the cells in the active growing region of the hair follicle. Now, here's where it gets technical. At a cellular level, testosterone encounters an enzyme called 5-alpha reductase and is converted to its usable form, dihydrotestosterone (DHT). In most areas of the body, this conversion is no big deal, as DHT has no real role in adult biological processes. But DHT does have a detrimental effect on two areas of the body: the prostate and hair follicles.

In the prostate (the prostates of *all* men, by the way, not just bald men), DHT causes the gland to swell, a condition known as benign prostatic hyperplasia (BPH). In its most minor forms, BPH can cause urinary difficulty when the prostate begins constricting the urethra. In advanced cases, it can lead to prostate cancer. BPH used to be curable only through expensive and painful surgery, until the discovery of finasteride, a 5-alpha reductase inhibitor that blocks testosterone from being converted to the hateful DHT. Remember that; it becomes important later.

The same conversion of testosterone to DHT that swells the prostate also causes hair follicles—but only in men who've inherited their father or mother's "baldness genes"—to miniaturize and produce increasingly wispy hair until eventually they are producing no hairs at all. Men with the genetic predisposition to baldness don't have more testosterone in their bodies (sorry, guys), but they do convert more of it to DHT in the scalp, thanks to higher levels of 5-alpha reductase. And men also have 50 percent more DHT receptor sites in the front part of their heads.

Finasteride, whether in its 5-milligram prostatic dosage (marketed as Proscar) or in its 1-milligram baldness dosage (marketed as Propecia), lowers DHT in the blood by about 70 percent.

Female pattern baldness—which consists of diffuse hair loss rather than the defoliation of whole regions of the scalp—is caused by a different mechanism, recent studies show. Unlike men, whose baldness begins just after puberty with the onset of testosterone production, most women who go bald won't see it until they're well into their fifties.

"It's an entirely different disease because it has nothing to do with testosterone," said O'Tar Norwood, a hair transplant pioneer who has recently devoted his attention to female baldness [http://www.hairclinic.com]. "That's why Propecia doesn't work on women."

Twenty percent of men at age twenty-five are already losing their hair. By age fifty, half the male population are. By age sixty, 75 percent are. With women, Norwood found, by age twenty-five, only 3 percent had lost hair. By age fifty, 16 percent had. By age eighty, 28 percent were balding.

Several new 5-alpha reductase inhibitors are making their way to the market, as well as a half dozen other promising treatments for baldness. New developments have been so swift that even the father of hair transplants sees that his services will soon no longer be needed.

"The day of medical control of all aspects of hair growth comes closer," Orentreich said recently.

*Chapter 3*

—

# "SHEER BUNCOMBE":
# THE SNAKE-OIL ERA

"Women's liberation will not be achieved until a woman can become paunchy and bald and still think that she's attractive to the opposite sex."

—EARL WILSON,
nightlife columnist, *New York Post*

In 1941, a Los Angeles doctor named Charles Alfred Jenson hung out the shingle of his new practice, a clinic devoted to baldness with the scientifically pleasing name the Scalp Institute.

As was permitted in those days, Jenson took out an advertisement in the local paper that detailed his "12-year investigation" into the causes of baldness and its potential redress. Unlike many shysters of the day, Jenson did not claim that hat wearing, dandruff or hot water caused baldness and he didn't overstate the success of the treatment he proposed, admitting that he could not "grow hair where hair roots have been lost."

But he held out the hope that bald men throughout the ages have yearned to hear: "The hair you have now can be saved."

Jenson was a harmless-looking fellow (though oddly inclined toward Hitler-style mustaches). The four-page brochure he handed to prospective patients was devoid of the era's transparent come-ons and slippery language. The cover was even adorned by the caduceus, the interlocking serpents that serve as the medical community's proud symbol.

True, the language was hopeful and the details vague, but there was something believable about Jenson's pitch.

"Baldness is cured by the gradual absorption of subcutaneous fat," he wrote in a pamphlet called "No Need Now to Lose Your Hair." "As absorption continues, the blood vessels become constricted, the blood supply to the scalp is increasingly reduced."

Jenson claimed that he had done actual autopsies on actual human bodies that revealed how follicles were "starved to death" because of constriction of blood vessels in the scalp.

But like all of the shadowy surgeons operating under the radar of federal and state authorities, very little was known about Jenson, an unmarried loner who lived in a fleabag hotel in a run-down Los Angeles neighborhood.

In the style of the times, Jenson stopped short of explaining his miracle cure for baldness—even as he was overtly stating its miraculousness. "The treatment requires only one sitting—one hour out of a lifetime and you can be rid of the threat of baldness." Nor would the good doctor explain his techniques without an office visit: "To be understood by the lay mind, it must be explained with the aid of anatomical drawings on hand in the office."

It all sounded so logical—but Jenson's miracle cure remains one of modern medicine's darkest moments. Only after an examination by Jenson (with the aid of those anatomical drawings, of course) did patients find out what they were in for: A mysterious clear substance Jenson called "pantine" would be injected with a six-inch needle directly into the tissue under the scalp. Jenson said that the injections would put some distance between the hair-bearing area of the scalp and the fatty layer below, where follicles die.

The patients had no way of knowing that "pantine" was really liquid wax—or that Dr. Jenson had the ethics of Dr. Mengele.

Yet his practice took off, further evidence that even in that supposedly modern era, men would jump at anything for the promise of restored hair. And then, as now, would-be patients were too intimidated by the medical professional in their midsts to question the doctor or ask to see successfully treated patients.

The American Medical Association started receiving requests for information on Jenson from curious potential customers about a year after the doctor set up shop.

The best repository of case studies of the era—millions of documents demonstrating the terrible, dangerous and illogical lengths to which men will go to overcome baldness—are housed in the AMA headquarters on North State Street in Chicago.

The case of Charles Alfred Jenson and the scores of patients he butchered is but one of thousands contained in the AMA archives, a small third-floor office that is officially known as the AMA's Historical Health Fraud and Alternative Medicine Collection. The documents span the prime "snake-oil" years, from the creation of the AMA's Bureau of Investigation in 1906 until the mid-1970s, long after the Food and Drug Administration's Pure Food and Drug Act (1906) and the subsequent Food, Drug and Cosmetic Act (1938) redefined what could and could not be done in the name of selling medicines or developing surgical techniques.

The documents are meticulously kept—scholars must make appointments and pay a fee just to get at them—and minutely indexed. Dozens of file folders offer painful glimpses into what passed for medicine in an earlier age.

Most file folders contain the historical record of a specific company, like the notorious "Thomas' System" (whose ads featured Zeppo Marx, most likely without his consent), or doctor, like Jenson. As you flip through each folder from the first page to the last, a pattern emerges: The files start out innocently enough, with a breathless, optimistic claim of efficacy and utility in the race to cure baldness ("I grew my own hair and I will grow yours," said the advertisement for Vreeland's Hairerbs in 1926), a positive newspaper article, perhaps some glowing testimonials (which could easily be bought from quasimedical, or even nonmedical, scam artists), a wave of hopeful-yet-concerned letters to the AMA from bald men or women seeking information before squandering their precious dollars on yet another pipe dream, and then letters of disgust as the dupes put their bad experiences on the record for AMA investigators. Very often there is also a paper trail left in the wake of government action, such as a mail fraud finding or a disciplinary hearing, against the company or doctor.

Those requests for information generally started pouring in a year after the appearance of the new product or technique, and the AMA, which was tracking thousands of shysters, typically responded to those initial letters claiming that it lacked specific information on this one company because there had not yet been enough requests to warrant a laboratory test on the product in question. But after ten or so letters, the Bureau of Investigation could usually reveal the results of their analysis: the products were always useless.

In Jenson's case, the AMA didn't know about the doctor until receiving a 1942 letter of query from Robert Richardson of West Los Angeles, who was contemplating going under Jenson's knife.

"Are these birds charlatans or have they got something on the ball?" Richardson asked, following a pattern of dubious hope that repeats in file after file. "One is naturally suspicious of anything hatched in Los Angeles, the nut capital of the world."

This being the organization's first contact with Jenson, the response from the AMA's Bureau of Investigation was weak: "We do not have any details as to the particular one-hour procedure. . . . We know of no scientific reports of such a procedure, and we believe it is reasonable to doubt the success of such a procedure in most, if not all, cases of baldness."

But Jenson's practice thrived, even as the AMA was receiving more and more queries about him and his $50, one-hour treatment. "We have no comment," the Bureau of Investigation wrote in 1946.

Finally, the walls of Jenson's Scalp Institute came tumbling down. Maimed and brutalized patients started alerting the authorities to Jenson's unethical practices.

"This man was giving a scalp treatment here which was supposed to prevent one from losing hair by cushioning the blood vessels from the constricting action of the scalp," patient Raymond Ettelson wrote to the AMA in 1947. "He injected a substance, believed to be similar to paraffin, and spread it all around the scalp. When I took the treatment he guaranteed that there would be no after-effects . . . except for discomfort for a couple of days. It is three months since my treatment and I have been suffering continuously from pain and swelling and have been unable to work. All my hair is falling out."

Ettelson claimed that other patients had been suffering the "after-effects" of Jenson's injection of paraffin—basically, liquid candle wax—under the scalp. Some were horribly disfigured when the material shifted, re-formed and hardened into subcutaneous bumps.

"This man definitely knew of the results of his treatment and yet continued to practice it which stamps him as a criminal," he continued. "Surgeons . . . say it is just about necessary to scalp a person to get the material out."

Ettelson became the point man in the preparation of a class-action suit against Jenson—but before the papers could be served, the doctor had skipped town. "The last information we had of him he was in Nevada on his way east, allegedly to New York."

The AMA response? *We had no idea he left Los Angeles.*

The magnitude of suffering meted out by Charles Alfred Jenson was slowly becoming clear. Ettelson wrote back to say that he was about to be operated on by a doctor to extract the hardened wax. "The whole scalp must be laid open," Ettelson wrote.

Others were not so lucky. At least one patient demanded that Jenson himself do the repair work. "For a long period of time, he kept coming to Jenson while the latter kept jabbing a needle into him. When this failed to produce results, Jenson subjected him to a brutal operation," Ettelson reported.

Harold Coar of Fort Wayne, Indiana, was never in such a serious state. A pilot with the air force, Coar was stationed in nearby Victorville, California, during World War II. Later, he flew in the Berlin airlift.

"He and some of the other flyboys were going bald and that went against their sense of beauty," Erie Coar, his widow, told me. "So they went to this Jenson for the procedure."

Coar was twenty-seven when he allowed his scalp to be subjected to Jenson's needle. A few years later, when he and his wife moved back to Fort Wayne, Coar noticed bumps under his skin. He wasn't in pain so much, but the bumps were so noticeable that he felt he had to do something about them. So in late 1947, he traveled to Chicago for an operation to remove the paraffin.

"He said it was like beeswax," Erie Coar recalled. "They had to literally scrape Harold's skull to get it all."

Afterward, the doctor who performed the surgery sent the AMA a sample of the wax for analysis and a description of what he witnessed under Coar's scalp: "The material was injected beneath Mr. Coar's scalp for the purpose of curing baldness. Since then there has been a gradual increasing swelling. . . . This morning, I aspirated the swelling and removed considerable light yellow, soft wax . . . and a considerable quantity of cloudy, reddish-brown fluid."

The AMA response? *Our lab is not set up to examine waxes.*

Thus relieved of his waxy buildup, Coar lived the rest of his life quietly as a corporate pilot, his widow said. "But for the rest of his life, he had an indentation in his skull where the wax had been."

With Jenson on the lam and no law-enforcement agency giving chase, one victim, John Bessor of Zelienople, Pennsylvania, tried a different tack. Bessor, who was an animator for Disney around the time he was "treated" by Jenson, took out an ad in the Los Angeles *Examiner* seeking to get in touch with other men who had been maimed by the doctor.

He got a response, amazingly, from Jenson himself asking Bessor for more information about his surgery "so I can consult my records. This is necessary as some refinements were made during the years I operated."

The letter had a New Orleans return address. Bessor wrote back to that address but never got an answer. When he wrote again, all he received was a nasty message saying that Jenson did not live there anymore.

"I never heard from the madman again," Bessor wrote.

But Bessor's ad produced a pouch of mail. John Davey of Burbank, a "fellow sufferer," wrote, "What saps we were! Gad, when I think of it, I feel like I must have been outta my mind." Davey was angry but was trying to get on with his life.

Bessor could not. "This ruiner of young men ought to be fully prosecuted," he wrote to the AMA in 1949. The AMA response: *It's not our job because Jenson isn't in the AMA.*

Bessor's disfigurement at the hands of Jenson—"the monster's inch-high humps [make] it impossible to be seen anywhere without a hat"—would be his obsession until he died. He abandoned his promising career at Disney—where he had worked on the 1942 movie *Bambi,* of all things—and moved back to his family farm in Pennsylvania, raising chickens and stewing in his own anger.

Still livid in 1955, he wrote again to the AMA demanding action: "For 12 years I have lived a veritable nightmare because of that 'queer' scalp monster, that fiend, that paranoidal, sadistic maniac. The fifty odd blaubs [*sic*] of paraffin he shot into my scalp (and in my blood stream, as well, I suppose) have caused me no end of growling scalp pains, day and night."

Comforted only by his bitterness and the support of his fellow victims, Bessor ascribed all manner of motivations to Jenson, from simple sadism to homoeroticism.

I now know that these disfiguring bumps were Jenson's cleverly thought out 'time bombs' to plague his victims in later years, possibly terminating in cancer. . . . I am pretty sure, now, that the man found in his six-inch needle a certain compensation for a flagging virility. In short, his needle was a symbol, and young *men* his victims. I have no doubt that, as he ran the needle along the skull, ejaculating blaubs [*sic*] of paraffin as he thrust, he was experiencing a weird kind of pleasure. Hideous thought, and to think that I must rue his vile raping till I die! I shall never forget his squeaky, high-pitched voice.

The last, single-sheet document in the two-hundred-page folder is, of course, a final letter from Bessor, sad to report that a Dr. Ruben

Chier had offered to remove the wax for $300—a sum that was too dear even for a man in agony.

"I don't know what to do," Bessor said, saying he could not afford the operation. "It has crippled my social life and ruined chances of marriage."

Still a young man when he wrote those words, Bessor's greatest torment was that he would live to see them come true.

"No, he never married," his sister-in-law Frances Bessor, who still lives in Zelienople, told me by phone. "He lived with his sister, who also never married, until he died a few years ago."

"By the time I got to know him [when Bessor had moved back from L.A.], he was a strange individual," added his nephew William Bessor, describing a "brilliant" man who was so fascinated by ancient Egypt that he would make replicas of famous mummies that were so good that he sold them to the Pittsburgh Museum. And William Bessor confirmed what his aunt suspected: The botched surgery ruined Bessor's life. "I never knew him to go out with women at all."

Frances Bessor described her brother-in-law with sadness about what happened to him and the obsession that it wrought. "He was an eccentric, but he was brilliant. Once he got on a topic, he never let it go. He was an extremely nice-looking man, but, you know, come to think of it, I never saw him without a hat on."

—

Has anything really changed? Jenson's level of brutality was unmatched, but his targeted wooing of the vulnerable and insecure remains a staple in the hair restoration industry.

In 1999, the State of New Jersey sued a company called United Microsystems—marketers of a hair replacement method it called Dermal Retention System—for allegedly defrauding "carefully targeted . . . vulnerable consumers [with] great psychological anxiety."

"Many men with thinning hair feel different, less attractive or less confident," the suit charged. "Defendants market their Dermal Retention System to these vulnerable consumers."

United Microsystems—which did not return my repeated calls for comment even as it tried to lure me as a customer when I called for more information about its product—has had a history with the State of New Jersey. In 1994, the state attorney general sued the company's precursor, International Cosmetics Labs, over a procedure that involved suturing a hairpiece directly into customers' heads—a procedure that is illegal.

The 1999 suit against United Microsystems alleges that the company fraudulently used fake before-and-after photos that appeared in ads in *Esquire* and *Muscle and Fitness* about a revolutionary "European Baldness Treatment." According to the allegations, the ads were nothing more than lies, using meaningless terms like "zero release factor," claiming that Dermal Retention "infuses hair filaments without surgical risks," that the process involves applying "small clusters of individual hair filaments," and that it "does not use a solid base hairpiece."

The problem? "Dermal Retention amounts merely to gluing a toupee to the scalp," the New Jersey attorney general's office charged. "As if their poor appearance was not enough, virtually every customer who has complained . . . reports that the UMS hair system quickly comes loose."

OK, so United Microsystems is no Charles Alfred Jenson, and no man was permanently disfigured. But the similarities between United Microsystems and the false cures of the past are clear: the same wildly hyperbolic claims of success, the same gloss of credibility lent by a "European" system, the same lies, the same unsatisfied customers.

Even the language used by United Microsystems' unsatisfied customers bears a close resemblance to John Bessor's agonized wails. All of the many people who testified against the company spoke of the humiliation of admitting their own vanity, the emotional drain of seeing hopes dashed and the anger at falling for the old bait-and-switch when they realized too late that the finished product on their heads did not match the picture-perfect company brochures.

One man described a preprocedure slide show that sounded exactly like Jenson's dog-and-pony presentation with the "anatomical drawings." Another mentioned that consent forms were signed only after the procedure was under way, another Jenson trick. Still another noticed that United Microsystems was deceptive about the actual substances used to affix the hairpiece to the head, another form of Jenson's mysterious "pantine." And everyone complained of spending thousands of dollars on lies.

"My wife commented that the netting was clearly visible," Anthony Cresci of New Jersey testified in the case against United Microsystems. "My wife also noticed a hard crusty ridge that encircled my head where the hairpiece ended. There are just no civil words to describe my hurt, humiliation, frustration and anger. I was physically and emotionally devastated when I realized what United Microsystems had done to me. . . . I look worse since the removal of the unit than before I started this whole process."

And like Bessor, Cresci concluded, "I feel extremely self-conscious about my appearance and frequently wear hats to cover up the damage done by United Microsystems."

As part of a settlement announced in July 2000, the company agreed to pay some $300,000 in fines, consumer restitution, and administrative and legal costs. Without admitting any wrongdoing, United Microsystems also agreed to change certain of its advertising and sales practices.

Yet as of this writing, United Microsystems' come-ons still adorn the pages of tabloid newspapers and national magazines: "New Revolutionary European Baldness Treatment Ends Baldness Now and Forever," the ad reads, promising essentially what was promised before the New Jersey settlement. "Dermal Retention . . . directly inserts hairs to scalp area safely and painlessly."

The United Microsystems brochures still tout a "four-hour procedure" to "infuse the Dermal Retention hair filaments," although customers still claim the procedure takes little longer than twenty minutes. And the brochure still denies the existence of a standard toupee base, showing instead hair filaments being individually woven into a man's existing hair. It remains unclear what, if anything, the settlement did except ring up some money for the State of New Jersey.

A century after some of the worst charlatanism and decades after federal legislation was supposed to end such abuse, shysters and cheats still ply their pernicious trade to the same kinds of frustrated, lonely, anxious men who are searching for an end to their misery. They find their victims with newspaper ads and woo them with overstated claims and mysterious, unverifiable success stories. Are they so different from the so-called snake-oil salesmen of the past?

Having flipped through thousands of pages at the AMA archives, I can tell you that the answer is no.

"The Secret of Conquering Baldness!" proclaimed a brochure written by the Koskott Laboratory in New York City in 1911. "The only practical book ever issued upon this subject."

As a historical example, Koskott—which was run by Edward J. Woods, one of the snake-oil era's most notorious shysters—provides a complete look at how such companies prospered in the era just before federal regulation.

In 1906, Congress passed the first of several important food and drug laws that required certain ingredients—alcohol, morphine, etc.—to be labeled, and made it illegal to make "false" or "misleading" claims. But the law did not cover cosmetics or medical devices. And a subsequent legal challenge encouraged the Supreme Court to weaken the law, making it more difficult to enforce, according to John Swann, historian for the Food and Drug Administration [http://www.fda.gov/cder/about/history/gallery/gallery1.htm].

"It was hard to enforce what was a 'misleading' or 'false' statement because the company could just say, 'Well, we *thought* it was true,' " Swann said.

Three decades would pass before Congress fought back, passing the Food, Drug and Cosmetic Act in 1938, which outlawed false therapeutic claims and gave the FDA some enforcement teeth. But in that thirty-two-year period, fake cures—like those by Koskott Laboratories—flourished.

The company's AMA file also begins with a harmless-sounding pitch. In this case, Koskott claimed that baldness was caused by a microscopic bacteria—the "dermodex folliculorum"—which invaded the scalp.

In case you haven't heard of the dermodex folliculorum, don't worry. It was, in fact, discovered "some years ago" by Dr. Gustav Simon, "a noted German specialist [who] proved to an absolute certainty that this parasite actually exists and thrives upon the scalps of those persons who are troubled with thinning and falling hair."

The pamphlet, of course, even included an artistic representation of what the folliculorum looked like under the microscope. As you can imagine, the dermodex folliculorum was depicted as a hideous, toothsome beastie, thick and black with sharp claws with which to grab on to your hair, and teeth with which to devour it.

"Perhaps you have heard people mention that they inherited baldness from their parents or grandparents," the pamphlet continued. "Perhaps you have the same notion. It is a mistake. There is no such thing as hereditary baldness. What has been inherited is the habit of using the same brush and comb as other members of the family and perhaps the habit of neglecting to clean these toilet requisites often."

Anticipating the prospective patient's next question, the brochure went on to explain that the reason children—who used the same "toilet requisites"—didn't contract baldness was because they were out in the sun a lot and didn't wear hats.

Naturally, dermodex folliculorum was contagious, "like typhoid fever, cholera, consumption or smallpox," the patient was told. "It reaches your scalp by means of a hair brush or comb that has been used upon the hair or scalp of another person. Or you may acquire one or several of the dermodex folliculorum by leaning against a cushion upon which the head of another has lain."

*Several?*

In case that wasn't scary enough, the seemingly scientific brochure trotted out another shadowy European expert, "Dr. Max Lasar of Germany," to inflict even more anxiety through wholly unverifiable "European" research. Dr. Lasar, the would-be patient was told, rubbed only two flecks of dermodex folliculorum–laced dandruff particles on the skin of an animal—and incited baldness within days! That the idiocy of the company's "research" was not clear to the thousands of bald men who forked over $1.12 per Koskott treatment is testimony to man's insuperable gullibility.

How could people not see through such charades as Koskott's "laboratory test"? "Our investigator in his laboratory put hairs from different heads into a solution containing the [Koskott formula]. These hairs remained four weeks, being tested in the meantime. In one case, the hair developed in strength 14 percent in one week. In four weeks, it had developed 31 percent."

The test is absurd: Hair is nothing but dead cells. Hair can't be "developed" in anything—especially after being removed from the follicle.

Yet tributes to the Koskott Treatment poured in—if you believe the company's propaganda. The treatment was even sanctioned by Dr. A. B. Griffiths, who was described as "a Ph.D., FRS and a member of the chemical societies of Paris and St. Petersburg." Again, just vague enough and just unverifiable enough to be plausible.

Griffiths wrote that he had "no hesitancy in giving the Koskott Treatment the high endorsement earned by the examination in these laboratories." Naturally he had no hesitancy; the AMA later revealed that "scientists" like Griffiths would sell such testimonials for $5 a pop.

The historical record is unclear what happened next. Koskott prospered for about a decade but then disappeared, overcome, perhaps, by the collective dissatisfaction of its customers.

That is the typical pattern of the shysters who flourished from the late 1800s to the 1930s, when real medicine and medical treatment were expensive. And not inconsequentially, the shysters were aided in their work because the price of shipping their products—and the cost of the glass bottles in which they came—had begun to drop dramatically in the late nineteenth century.

In 1920, Forst's Original Bare-to-Hair entered the vast market of hair growth products claiming, like so many others, that it was a "scalp fertilizer and germicide" that "destroys the cause of all hair trouble [and] destroys the germ which is the cause of most hair trouble."

Doctors, barbers and even the director of public welfare from Lynchburg, Virginia, started writing the AMA almost immediately. Even without analyzing the solution, the association was skeptical. "Neither can we say that the 'before and after' pictures in the circular you send impress us greatly," the AMA's Propaganda Department, as it was then known, wrote back to the concerned public servant in Lynchburg. "The gentleman in the 'after' pictures merely looks as though his head was dirty." Later, the AMA upgraded its attack. "The statement that this stuff 'will grow hair on a bald head' is a preposterous falsehood."

The product disappeared around 1930.

Outright lies and an uneducated public were the currency of the snake-oil salesmen. When viewed in the aggregate, it's easy to see the extent of the deception. But each of the very short-lived companies told a different lie and peddled a different concoction.

The products also invariably played on the paranoia and anxiety of vulnerable bald men. Almost every company, however, even the ones that made the most outrageous claims, would intentionally admit that its product was not 100 percent effective.

When you think about it, the strategy was bizarre, asking men to believe in the company because the company was admitting its product didn't always work.

"Will Formula BX97 do as much for you? It is impossible to say 'Yes.' It is equally out of the question to say 'No,' " the brochure for Helois Humbert's product asked and then answered (vaguely). "All we say is that Formula BX97 has worked wonders for others. It may do the same for you."

And of course, the product—which was later found to consist solely of water, alcohol and a tiny amount of pilocarpine hydrochloride—was made from an exotic "South American shrub which has the unusual property of stimulating hair growth."

That's one of the common themes that runs throughout the history of fake cures, according to Albert Kligman, a dermatologist at the University of Pennsylvania and something of a hair historian. "These products share the following similarities: 1, they come in many forms, encompassing chemical and physical treatments. 2, they are medically unsound and unproved. And, 3, they usually cost a lot of money and are offered with supreme confidence in the outcome (money-back guarantees)."

Kligman also observed that the products tended to create a false exoticism—like those that were "discovered in the jungles of the Far East"—and were almost always comprised of substances so grotesque, hideous and unappealing that "they must be sure to work."

When he wrote that, Kligman was speaking of the ancient "cures" for baldness—such as the Roman technique of smearing hippo fat or the Egyptian technique of turning the charred remains of domesticated mice into a salve—but his words were just as fitting for America in the early part of this century.

In 1921, for example, the Aymes Company of New York City marketed the Dijiman Hair Drill as "the best treatment for the hair that money can buy." The product, which turned out to be nothing more than a powdered shampoo, was marketed with a lie: "Hair is formed from a fluid that Nature has separated from the blood," the company literature stated. "This fluid is an oil that is deposited in the root of the hair."

A decade later, Thomas Kridos, claiming that "the pressure of a hat-band" could block the follicles from getting "life-giving blood," marketed the Kridos System, which had, he claimed, won awards at several international expositions, including the "Exposition Internationale Palais Des Fêtes et Des Beaux-Arts Et Parc De La Boverie" in 1928.

"As for the various grand prizes and medals of honor that are awarded at so-called international expositions, they are merely a subject for sardonic laughter," the AMA wrote. Products such as the Kridos System "are, as a rule, sheer buncombe."

But exoticism was the rule of the day. In 1933, Adna Hall marketed a product called Lotta Lox, which she claimed was a "plant leaf product of South America." When a government chemist analyzed the product, it was found to be nothing more than glycerin, rose water and mullein, "a common plant which is found growing along the roadside and in the woods."

That same year, a company called Alwin Products took out ads to tout their new product, Ambergren. As for many useless products, the Alwin company invented an elaborate tale, complete with faraway lands, bizarre local customs and heroic scientists.

The story had it that in 1919, an "ex-Army officer and scientist on one of his exploring expeditions to the Far East noticed that the natives of various Far Eastern countries had wonderful hair." The secret? "Their Teachers and Priests supply them with what the natives call 'Bal-Dava' (meaning hair medicine) which they use religiously."

But the ex-army officer couldn't, of course, merely walk off with some of this miracle Bal-Dava. No, this secret wasn't easy to come by: "They respect this secret as they do the idols of worship and guard it against discovery. [But] after many disappointments and much discouragement, the scientist, through a stroke of good luck, was able to discover the secret of this age-old hair medicine."

Upon returning to America, the scientist replicated the small quantity of Bal-Dava and rechristened it Ambergren (what, the fake name "Bal-Dava" wasn't good enough? They had to invent another fake name?).

Ambergren was, according to the AMA, more "buncombe."

Scams were often far more elaborate than merely peddling an inert product to a desperate man. A great deal of clever publicity also went into the marketing, which is one reason the era is viewed today with a mixture of genuine horror and winking delight right out of a P. T. Barnum pitch (not surprisingly, Barnum himself briefly peddled a baldness "cure" to the 1,440 suckers he estimated were born every day). With so many products on the market, inventors and their publicists had to think big in order to land favorable or even unfavorable media attention.

In 1916, Georgia O. George was hauled before San Francisco judge Morris Oppenheimer on charges that her "Hair-A-Gain" mixture was a fraud because it claimed it could "grow hair on an absolutely bald head."

Naturally, the press had been tipped off to the court appearance so George defended herself by telling the judge, "That is not a misstatement, Your Honor. That can be done."

The judge responded, "Show me," and, according to the San Francisco *Call,* George responded, "With pleasure." She then was invited back into chambers to apply "Hair-A-Gain" to the judge's head.

According to the paper, "From now on, the judge's bald spot will be watched with considerable interest, while the sporting element about the Hall of Justice is preparing to make a book [set odds] on the result of the treatment."

The news was picked up around the country, but the media moved on to other topics. So when Judge Oppenheimer finally issued his ruling, no paper covered it, giving George what she wanted: the lingering impression that she had won.

She stayed in business until the late 1920s.

A few years after George's success in the courts, Jules Ferond was cited for violating the sanitary code in the city of New York because his potion claimed to "positively grow hair" yet did not. The company was facing a $100 fine, but ended up making far more of that back in publicity.

Before Magistrate Alexander Brough, Ferond, who had originally developed the product to grow hair on his beloved dogs, testified that his product worked—and then called as witnesses many "customers" who testified to its efficacy. Brough didn't buy it and levied the full $100 fine. A few weeks later, however, the hardly chastened Ferond took out large ads in major papers around the country under the headline "Swore in Court that Ferond's Grows Hair!"

The ads recounted the testimony of the supposedly happy supposed customers, most if not all of whom had been paid off. "Their testimony is part of the Court Records of the City of New York, and marks an important development in the history of dermatology," the ad stated. It left out, however, what the court records show: "A number of persons . . . gave testimony to the effect that they had used this hair-grower and that it had not promoted the growth of their hair."

*The New York Times,* covering the all-day trial, added that "it was noticeable that those who testified had no considerable amount of hair. One man said that he had been totally bald for years and that after six applications of this hair tonic a slight floss had appeared on his scalp."

Ferond's hair tonic consisted solely of petroleum jelly, alcohol, water, saponifiable oil, salicylic acid, balsam of peru and perfume. Ferond could not grow hair, but he knew what to say in court.

In 1932, the makers of Hairmore struck gold with a seemingly indestructible sales pitch, claiming that the product had been invented by a Jesuit priest at Gonzaga University named James Gilmore.

The company claimed that Gilmore, who was said to be head of the school's science department and "one of the country's leading blood chemists," had invented the product to comfort a student who had picked up the unfortunate moniker of "Baldy" and was constantly being taunted by his fellow students.

And, being a Jesuit who had taken a vow of poverty, naturally Gilmore wasn't in it for the money. In fact, manufacture of Hairmore, according to company brochures, "is done by a group of deaf persons in Spokane, Washington. This opportunity was given them by Father Gilmore to provide for their livelihood." Profits were plowed back into the school.

Despite the fact that the AMA put out the word that "James A. Gilmore is quite unknown to scientific medicine," Hairmore had a long run before crashing under the weight of too many unsatisfied customers.

Sometimes the shysters got sold some snake oil themselves. In 1954, a Scottish doctor by the name of John Kelvin wrote in the *British Medical Journal* that several of his patients grew hair after being treated with Roniacol, a blood pressure medication made by Hoffman-LaRoche, one of the leading drug companies in the world.

It sounded so legit—hey, it sounds like Rogaine!—that the mainstream press jumped all over the *BMJ* report. "Scotch Doc Tells Hair-Raising Tale," read one headline.

The American Medical Association tried to throw cold water on the finding, reminding that at best, the only hair anyone had ever been able to grow on a bald head had been fuzz. And a Roche company spokesman said, "We have made no claims for Roniacol as a hair growth promoter."

"Hey, Baldy! Don't Let This Go to Your Head," reported the Chicago *Daily News* after the comments by Roche and the AMA.

But the word was out and Kelvin found himself inundated by bald men seeking treatment. He wasn't used to this kind of thing, the sudden commercialization of his practice. But someone else was.

Kelvin was immediately contacted by L. R. Akers, proprietor of the Akers' Hair and Scalp Clinics, who wooed the Scottish doctor with plans to join forces and create a "new scientific approach" to treating baldness. Kelvin, perhaps not realizing—or perhaps not caring—that, in America, the Akers name was synonymous with hucksterism, agreed to join him as a "research director."

Thus began Akers's massive advertising scheme, ads that featured some of the early press coverage and, of course, a glowing letter from Kelvin explaining that he was disbanding his clinic in Glasgow to join the Akers' Clinic "after long deliberation and exhaustive investigation."

The ads were in all the papers, but, as they say, the check was still in the mail. No contract was ever sent to Kelvin. And when a reputable hospital tried to repeat Kelvin's experiments, this time using the Akers formulation of it, it was able to grow only some light fuzz on some patients.

"It's going to be a big disappointment to thousands," said a spokesman for the hospital in Stoke Mandeville, England. "But there you are. It was worth a try."

Reports started coming back from patients. In one letter to the AMA, a client described a visit to an Akers clinic, which was situated in an "expensively furnished suite of rooms in [a] very modern office building."

An Akers representative did the examination, complaining that the patient had "waited too long" before coming to see him.

"He began to run a stick through my hair, all the while murmuring to himself and 'tsk-tsking,' " the patient explained. "He said my scalp was clogged and explained the condition with the aid of the anatomical chart on the wall, accompanying the explanation with a lecture on the anatomy and physiology of the hair. It was all very interesting, but quite meaningless and hardly accurate."

The patient was told that the "treatments" would cost a total of $250, plus $15 for "special cleaning materials and hair brush."

The AMA's opinion about the Akers' Hair and Scalp Clinics? "It is our impression that the 'scalp' part of it refers to the customers' pocketbooks."

In a subsequent ethics hearing back in Scotland, Kelvin said he was shocked—shocked?—to learn that the Akers clinics were "a mirage" and that he was "dealing with crooks and profiteers."

He said that he had scribbled his initial report to the *British Medical Journal* because he thought "it might technically interest a few doctors." He explained that bald men from all over the world sent him checks, which he returned uncashed. He maintained that he thought Akers was a reputable doctor.

The passage of the federal Food, Drug and Cosmetic Act in 1938, which created the Food and Drug Administration and set up new restrictions on the development and sale of cures, was the beginning of the end for the slick shysters of this bizarre era in American medical history.

Empowered by the act, by the 1940s, the federal government stepped up its efforts to arrest the growth of the snake-oil sellers, typically by finding the companies guilty of mail fraud because they used the U.S. Postal Service to ship their fraudulent products and receive their ill-gotten revenues.

Postal Service files are filled with such cases, which follow the familiar pattern: a complaint by a duped member of the public, an anonymous order placed by a postal investigator, an analysis of the product by a government chemist, a finding that the product contained inert ingredients much more likely to buff your car than grow hair on your head, a hearing at which the maker of the product defended its efficacy, and a finding of fraud by a Postal Service hearing officer.

But most of the companies were not companies at all, just mom-and-pop perpetrators who could easily reinvent themselves as a new company with a different name and a different (in name only) product that could avoid Postal Service scrutiny for another few years.

Edward Hidden had an appropriate last name and a typical way of doing business. Cited with mail fraud in the 1930s for a fake obesity medication, he merely reconfigured his "laboratory" to fabricate Nuhair, a substance that "will produce a full growth of hair on bald-headed persons—even those as bald as a billiard ball."

Escaping detection for years, Hidden was finally summoned before the Postal Service in 1941. His Nuhair consisted of alcohol, castor oil, kerosene and a drop or two of betanaphthol.

A year later, a guy named Harry Hitter suddenly came out with a product called "Growhair." When the Postal Service caught up with Hitter, it discovered that Growhair was remarkably similar to Nuhair: alcohol, kerosene, castor oil and a touch more of betanaphthol.

Hitter, who had formerly sold vacuum cleaners, was hit with an investigation for fraud.

In every file is another story:

• Johnson's Miracle Hair Grower (1942): The Postal Service tested some and discovered that it consisted solely of "glycerin and mushroom extractives" with benzoates as a preservative. When the creator of the miracle cure, Charles Johnson, was called to testify, the court records show that he claimed that "while doing work in a garage, he heard a voice telling him that baldness could be cured. He immediately began a search for something and once, while out walking, he looked down and saw a mushroom, which he thereafter chose as the active ingredient with which to cure baldness." Johnson, an electrician from Portland, Oregon, acknowledged under oath that the mushrooms were nothing more than "the common edible variety" and that he picked them up at his local market.

• Renucel (1952): The Postal Service chemist found that this product consisted of nothing more than "castor oil with a trace of combined iodine." Maker Germaine Urban employed a novel strategy at her hearing, claiming that even if the product didn't grow hair, her job was to pretend that it did. "Faith and hope play a part in the restoration of hair," she testified. Her hearing officer, Robert Piper, took a far grimmer view of Urban's attempt to sell a placebo: "A psychological theory that a person with belief that [Urban's] product will regrow hair will have better results than a person without such beliefs [despite] established medical facts to the contrary does not appear to warrant extended discussion." Piper ruled it a fraud.

• H.H.L. Scalp Rub (1948): La-San Laboratories, based in Yeadon, Pennsylvania, was run by Max Levinsky, a pharmacist who claimed that since 1925 he had been studying to "solve the mysteries of different diseases which the doctors could not correct." For baldness, Levinsky sold a rub (for $10, no less) that would "stimulate the growth of hair. Yes—today you can be relieved from baldness [with] this new war formula." New war formula? The Postal Service found that the formula was nothing more than petroleum jelly, water and ichthyol, which may be some kind of fish extract. On cross-examination, Levinsky admitted that he used his product to treat his own baldness and that he "had a little bit more hair now than I had when I started" and claimed his head was only one-eighth bald. But according to the postal trial examiner Daniel Kelly, Levinsky was optimistic. "The respondent while testifying was approximately 12 feet from me, and from my position, it appeared that at least one-fourth, if not one-third, of the top of the respondent's head was bald. . . . He claimed that he had grown hair after using his preparation for two years on the part of his head which appeared to be bald, but he admitted that this hair could not be seen from a distance." Levinsky was cited for fraud, but not because he peddled a bad drug, but a bad cosmetic, which was also illegal. "A man purchasing a cure for baldness is not seeking anything to improve his health, but only to improve his appearance. . . . Apparently, the only type of hair which might appear on a bald spot after the use of the respondent's product is the type of fuzz or down which was on the respondent's bald spot at the hearing and could not be seen at a distance of 12 feet. This is not the type of hair a purchaser of his product would reasonably expect from the advertising claims of the respondent."

The U.S. Postal Service is still empowered to prosecute fraudulent companies as long as customers use the mails to buy the product or the companies use the mails to send it. In this day of telephone transactions and purchases sent by FedEx, the Postal Service is not as busy as it once was. And, perhaps, the days of the snake-oil salesmen are passing.

"Those kinds of cases aren't as common anymore," said Lisa Martin, chief of consumer protection for the Postal Service. "I'd imagine that with Rogaine and Propecia, the demand for quack products has decreased."

Or it just could be that the Internet has become the new means of relieving desperate men of their cash. Dozens of websites hawk a variety of baldness "cures," always tailored to the latest scientific development.

"I remember one site was selling a product that, it claimed, worked just like Rogaine," said Ken Washenik, director of dermatopharmacology at New York University. "Then, when Propecia came out and everyone knew that dihydrotestosterone was the culprit, suddenly the website changed: 'Lowers DHT!' The product didn't change, but the website did."

Absurdity continues today all over the world. In Japan, consumers are advised to buy a special brush and hit their scalps two hundred strokes daily (true to a culture obsessed with exactitude, the brush automatically keeps track of the number of blows).

The product, like so many American versions from the early part of this century, may have a role in improving blood flow to the scalp—but it is hardly marketed as credible science.

"Japanese men are beaten at work, they are beaten at home, and beating makes strong men!" Like the AMA before him, Albert Kligman called this "irresistible humbug."

"Quackery thrives on ignorance," he concluded.

Always has, always will.

# Chapter 4

—

# THE RUG MEN

"Nothing is more unsightly than a bald man covered with hair."
—MARTIAL (c. 40–103), Roman poet

In the back corner of a styling room at the New York hairpiece emporium Penthouse for Hair Recovery is a full-scale photograph of owner Elliot Nonas that is as great a reminder of the 1970s than any time capsule buried in the cornerstone of a school.

The black-and-white photo shows Nonas decked out in decade-perfect tennis whites—Lacoste polo shirt, polyester shorts, knee-high sweat socks, Puma sneakers—holding aloft a Wilson wood racquet.

Ah, but there's one more element of the picture that dates it to the Disco Era. On top of Nonas's head is a crown of curly hair so thick, so lush that it looks as if John McEnroe's hair—not the individual follicles, mind you, but the entire scalp—had been surgically removed and repositioned on Nonas's head, sweatband and all.

That crown, that pelt, that Elysium of hair, was a toupee of Nonas's creation. He called it "The Headhugger."

The priceless photo is a classic in the way that it explains, in one quick glance, how (and, more important, *why*) the age of free love came crashing down under the weight of its own self-indulgence.

But what is even more important is how this image—"The Headhugger"!—remains the snapshot that flashes into the public consciousness whenever the word "toupee" is uttered, even though we are thirty years from the Headhugger's heyday.

Maybe it is for this reason—a cautionary reminder of a decade of shaggy excess in the form of a grotesque, white-man Afro—that Nonas keeps the photo around at all.

"We knew it looked like shit even back then!" Nonas told me. "But this was the seventies and people wanted hair, hair, hair! The Headhugger was enormous! It covered the whole head. It had a stainless-steel band across the top that held it against your head. I used to set off metal detectors at airports!"

If it sounds strange to hear a toupee man mock his own product—which he still sells, by the way, to men who don't know better or don't *care* to know better—you don't know Elliot Nonas.

Nonas—who proudly wore the Headhugger but now opts for a modern, almost undetectable model—is one of the last of a dying breed of rug men. Where there was once shame, Nonas and others gave bald men the faith and support to do what men simply did not do back then—wear what is essentially a knitted skullcap of someone else's hair.

Even today, years after the toupee industry rose, crashed in a field of public ridicule and rose again (albeit more quietly this time), Nonas's Penthouse for Hair Recovery retains a fifties frat-house feel that fully reflects its owner's proud yet self-effacing spirit. As if this were a real barbershop—you know, an old-time barbershop where you smoked while you waited for the head barber—Nonas provides free coffee and girlie magazines (and he calls them that) on every table. And on Saturday mornings, there's even a free buffet of bagels and eggs so customers can stop by for a collegial pat on the back from their proud head coach, to compare notes or to "lie about their conquests," even if they're not due for their regular, six-week cleaning and regluing.

Nonas has created, as he summed it up in an ad a few years ago, "The Best Little Hair House in New York."

There really are only two businesses in which a character like Elliot Nonas could thrive and, fortunately for him, they are at root the same business. Before he started making hairpieces, Nonas was a somewhat important figure on Madison Avenue, cranking out ad copy for a variety of clients, including Grolier's Encyclopedia ("Wanna read a good book?"), the Irish Tourist Office ("The Last Angry Bargain!") and Faberge cosmetics (one of Nonas's perfume commercials, featuring a woman in a slip and a stud at her bedside, won a Clio even though it was turned down by CBS "because it was too raunchy").

But when he started doing print ads for a friend's toupee company ("Baldness: You can stop it through castration. If that's too drastic, read on"), he started down an inexorable road to becoming a "wearer," as the term goes—and, eventually, the owner.

For toupees, that was a long but vital journey. Like hair transplant surgeons who still did large-plug for years after superior techniques had been perfected, the toupee industry clung to the Headhugger and monstrosities like it for too long because the money was too good. Nonas was selling thousands of them, he says, at $500 a pop, "which was a lot of money back then."

"The seventies were a very special time," the eighty-five-year-old Nonas says. "If there was an Internet then, I'd have sold Headhuggers directly to the customer and I'd be sitting on my yacht right now in Positano with hookers on both arms." (They'd have to be hookers if Nonas had kept wearing that Headhugger.)

Today Nonas knows better. He still cherishes his Positano/hooker fantasy, but when a customer comes in and requests a Headhugger, Nonas screams at him, "You'll look like a freak in that!"

Harvey Russo, one of Nonas's competitors, sees it all the time, too.

"A sixty-year-old guy came in here the other day and pulls out an ad from Camel cigarettes, points to the guy with all the hair and says, 'I want to look like him,' " recalls Russo, owner of Top Priority, a hairpiece salon in Manhattan. "I turned him down. I told him to find someone else. He's going to look like a clown. I don't need that and my industry doesn't need that."

Russo says he told Burt Reynolds the same thing, but Reynolds insisted on the full head of hair look—you remember, the one that made him a *Smokey and the Bandit* laughingstock rather than the Oscar-worthy star of *Deliverance.*

"He wanted it thick and curly and no gray," Russo says. "You could not talk him out of it."

And some still want that Headhugger look today. "It's mostly older men who've always worn the big models and complain that they don't feel as comfortable with the newer, thinner toupees," Nonas says.

Selling ads or selling hair, Elliot Nonas is still doing the same thing: image making.

"I was in advertising for years," says Nonas, who would later do Liberace's hair. "I was the top guy. I made a million and lost a million and made a million again. But this is so much more gratifying. I take a bald guy and I give him back his confidence. He comes in a wallflower and he leaves here a guy who's hitting on all the broads."

This is a persistent theme you hear from all the rug men, especially the ones who prospered during the sexual revolution, an age of such freedom, we are told, when even fat men, ugly men and men wearing the Headhugger were enjoying the company (among other things) of attractive, free-spirited women.

But not if they were bald.

Sy Sperling knows that firsthand (or is that first *head?*). As founder of the Hair Club for Men—yes, he's also a client, as his late-night infomercials constantly remind us—Sperling is the living embodiment of the psychological trauma that occurs when a man goes bald.

Sperling was only twenty-seven when he started losing his hair—and with it his self-confidence. It wasn't long before he started gaining weight, he says, and withdrawing from social situations.

Transplants were available, but they were primitive in those days and Sperling says he did not even consider them. "And I would not wear a toupee," he adds. "In those days, a young guy would not wear a toupee. You just wouldn't do it."

Fortunately for Sperling, he happened to go bald just as a new type of hairpiece—the "hair *weave*"—was being rolled out. Instead of a toupee, which was taped onto the scalp (or, in some nefarious cases, laced through cylinders of skin that had been taken from your abdomen and sewn into your scalp to function as a sort of belt loop), the new weave hairpieces were sewn into a braid of a man's own side hair.

For Sperling, this made all the distinction in the world. He wouldn't be wearing a toupee, which men typically removed at night and stored on a head-shaped wooden block on their dresser, but a weave, which could remain on the head all the time. The change, as he describes it, was immediate.

"I lost thirty pounds and went to a singles weekend at Grossinger's in the Catskills," Sperling tells me as we chat in a conference room at the Hair Club headquarters in Boca Raton, Florida. "It was amazing. I had my confidence back and I was getting girls' phone numbers even as I was on line to check in. I left that weekend with a dozen numbers and I slept with two or three women while I was up there. It was phenomenal. And that's why I can say I absolutely, positively believe in this product, ten million percent."

On his website [http://www.hairclub.com], Sperling is even more hyperbolic: "There's nothing like self-fulfillment of one's passion to drive one to make a better mousetrap. Just as the Wright brothers may have enjoyed jumping off cliffs with giant gliders for the sheer feeling of ecstasy, it led them to develop the first airplane. I feel that my passion is similar."

Pictures from the era show the hairpiece-wearing Sperling as an attractive young guy. That he would walk out of Grossinger's with a diminished sperm count and a bolstered black book is not surprising at all.

"Sometime between the Pill and AIDS, there was Sy," says Mike Smith, a spokesman for Sperling's Hair Club for Men, referring to his boss's sudden success with the ladies.

But how do you explain Harvey Russo?

Russo tells similar stories of toupee-aided sexual conquests, but the picture of him on the wall of his office, while just as much a timepiece as Nonas's tennis shot, jars you like that recurring dream where you're taking a French final having not attended even one class all semester.

There's Russo, circa 1980, with a veritable helmet of curly black hair, standing in front of a *Today* show weather map with Willard Scott, who was not only the *Today* show forecaster, but also a Russo customer. With a thinning, gray toupee appropriate for his age, Scott looks great. With his Jew-fro of fake Headhugger-like hair, Russo looks like he just walked out of his own bar mitzvah.

"Even that guy got laid in the 1970s," Russo says, pointing to himself in the picture.

Part of the cause for disbelief is that the hairpieces being made today resemble those thick floor mats of yesteryear in no way except that they both cover the bald scalp. You would not know it from the image of toupees in the popular imagination (think of that episode of *Seinfeld* when bald agonist George Costanza gets a disastrous hairpiece or the time on *LA Law* when Brackman's brand-new toupee—which was made by Russo, by the way—falls off in front of a girl he's trying to impress), but we are living in a true Golden Age of Hairpieces.

Just pick up one of Nonas's old Headhuggers and compare it to the salt-and-pepper wig he wears today, which is detectable only if you notice that the gray hair sprinkled throughout doesn't perfectly match Nonas's own faded color. (That's because gray toupee hair—even in a human-hair toupee—is typically made of yak hair, which does not fade.) But that's nit-picking.

Where the old Headhugger piece had hair on top of hair on top of hair on top of a sweat-retaining cloth mesh, today's piece has a fraction of the hair atop a thin, breathable nylon mesh that's see-through when it lays against your flesh. When the hair is parted, you actually see the bald man's natural scalp, just as you do on a "normal" man's head.

Modern toupees start in the same place: the fitting room. Where once a cast of a man's head was made with plaster of Paris—a messy process that turned off plenty of potential customers—now a man will sit in a barber chair while the stylist covers his head with industrial Saran Wrap, the kind found in delicatessens all over the country. The wrap creates a shiny helmet, the plastic equivalent of a chrome dome.

The client then bunches up the excess wrap around his ears and pulls the handfuls of plastic—they resemble pigtails—while the stylist draws his hairline in blue wax pencil.

The Saran Wrap makes the perfect fit, but it won't retain its shape, so the man's plastic-wrapped head is then covered with longitudinal pieces of regular Scotch tape. And that's that.

The ensuing half-football-shaped "mold" is then sent to the factory, most of which are in the Far East today, along with a detailed instruction form that tells the factory whether the toupee gets a left part, right part, center part or something called a "pompadour freestyle," what type of curl to apply, how dense the hair should be and where it should be thinned out, how short it should be cut and what color goes where.

Six weeks later, the finished product comes back. If hair transplant surgeons are playing God, toupee makers are God's stylist. Properly glued—or taped, if you don't plan to wear it when you sleep, swim or shower—the toupee is almost undetectable. It can't be called a Headhugger. It can't even be called a rug.

"That's why I call it 'The Virtual Reality,' " Nonas says. Such a model costs $1,350 and will last about eight months if you wear it all the time.

Of course, not every toupee is a custom job—and shopping for a toupee is not typically an exercise in high fashion. Even though custom toupees can run $2,000, they are rarely sold with the kind of refinement one would expect, say, when buying a really expensive suit.

For Nonas, that's intentional. The idea is not to build up this product into something it is not. It is merely an article of clothing that gets taped to your head; it is not a new life.

But elsewhere the sale of toupees lacks Nonas's back-slapping salesmanship and honesty. Just search the Internet or the Yellow Pages and you'll be amazed at the artless way most off-the-rack toupees are sold today.

Most premade wigs are the same no matter where you purchase them. But each company makes an almost comical attempt to distinguish itself. The result is anything but distinguished.

At World of Wigs, an Atlanta toupee retailer, men can choose from toupee styles ranging in price from $225 to $350, ranging in names from the absurd to the moronic and ranging in style from slightly noticeable to "Hey, is that a *Hard Day's Night* wig you have on?"

Your choices include:

"The Jason" ($225): It's described as "casual for today's look," but the picture next to it makes it seem as though you are wearing a porcupine—a nice-looking porcupine, mind you—on the front of your head.

"The Ricardo" ($250): This thick helmet of hair features "reinforced hair pads [and] natural recession at front hairline with soft material for comfort all around." Judging by the picture, it should be called "The TV Weatherman (circa 1985)."

"The Kirk" ($250): Whoever said the rock band A Flock of Seagulls wasn't going to make a comeback obviously never saw this stunning hairpiece, inspired by the worst follicular offenses of 1980s rock. This "bi-level" cut is left long in the back, so that wings of hair fall down behind your ears, just like Charlie Sheen's in *Ferris Bueller's Day Off.*

"The Senator" ($295): If Gore Vidal designed a toupee, this would be the one. This silver-gray mix is "hand-tied" with a left side part and a "mesh center." We all know that members of Congress someday want to be senators, but how many are sporting "Senators" right now?

"The Tommy" ($350): This one could also be called "The One-Piece" for the astounding manner in which it covers your head in a shag dome straight out of the German postpunk techno movement. Long sideburns, which look almost like handlebars on this horrendous wig, complete the Devo-esque look of this modern Headhugger.

Of course, anyone wearing a toupee like that isn't interested in hiding the fact that he's wearing a toupee in the first place. Even in the probably retouched photos on the World of Wigs website, you can see that this is not high-quality merchandise. You can observe the thin line where the toupee meets the natural hair, discern a faint difference in the color between the hairpiece and the existing hair and flat out see where a patch of the toupee's straight hair meets a natural curl.

All toupees are noticeable in this way, but a good one is as close to undetectable as possible by today's science.

How did we get from there—from the universal contempt for a shoddy, unnatural product—to here? First, toupees needed boosters. And with his background in advertising, Elliot Nonas came to understand that this was to be his most important role.

Not that there was a career track for rug making. Nonas studied journalism at the University of Georgia and wrote articles for the local paper. By the time he graduated, he got an offer for a job as copy boy at a new national newsmagazine in New York called *Time*. It was a good, get-in-on-the-ground-floor offer, but Nonas (idiot!) turned it down.

"What did I know?" he says today. "I thought it was beneath me! I'd been published in the Athens *Daily News!*"

So he went into advertising. Years later a friend said he was going to buy a chain of hairpiece shops and wanted the bald Nonas to invest and then do the advertising. And he needed another favor.

"He wanted me to go to one of the shops and check them out because I was bald," Nonas recalls. "This was 1967. This was not the kind of thing that was done in those days. It wasn't acceptable to wear a toupee. That was only for actors or jerks, not Elliot Nonas! Elliot Nonas wearing a toupee? Never!"

Nonas was so nervous about even walking into the store that he put it off for two days. Finally he went into the shop and gave his approval of his friend's purchase. Now he was part owner of a toupee shop.

"So I had to start wearing a hairpiece because I couldn't keep telling the customers that my piece was in the cleaners," he says. But Nonas was still just an absentee owner, continuing to build his advertising business and stopping in at the toupee shop only occasionally.

But then, he says, he "became disenchanted" with the ad business. Whatever those words mean, Nonas isn't saying. Maybe there were some genuine problems with the industry or perhaps it's spin—maybe he just got squeezed out by younger talent reviving a stodgy, gray-flannel industry—but Nonas suddenly found himself the no-longer-absentee owner of a chain of toupee shops.

He bought out his coowners and renamed the place Penthouse for Hair Recovery, although the connection to the men's magazine of the same name is solely spiritual. At times Nonas has advertised in the magazine, but there's no other connection save the name, the general enthusiasm for lust of any kind and the fact that *Penthouse* once published a Nonas-penned poetic tribute to defecation, which Nonas proudly displays in his waiting room.

Nonas conceived of his Penthouse as the bald man's clubhouse it is today, complete with his "erotic" poetry on the walls and in the quarterly "Penthouse Papers" newsletter he publishes as the official organ of the toupee-wearing world.

"The Penthouse Papers" is filled with schmaltz, old stories, editorials, poems and bitter tirades against everything from bad toupees to Rudy Giuliani's and Sam Donaldson's bad comb-overs—"Why would two intelligent and celebrated men opt for a comb-over to hide their hair loss rather than accepting their baldness (as did Koch) or opting for some kind of hair replacement or transplants (as did Hugh Downs)?" Nonas asked.

"We're angry and we want you to be angry," Nonas wrote after another TV show featured a star whose toupee fell off. "We know and you know that a bonded system can't be pulled off without the same effort that would be required to yank out a handful of natural, growing hair. . . . Sure, you've seen it on TV, the stupid inspiration of untalented writers who think it's funny. Well, it ain't!"

And naturally there's heaping portions of Nonas's poems, most of which are paeans to an unrequited love, like this passage from a poem à clef that references the poet Dowson: "Ah, would that I could act as Dowson, faithful in his fashion / But for the nonce, Cynara is my one and only passion / Like Dowson, I am sore beset with love that's unrequited / Perhaps some day she'll say 'Let's fuck' and say it uninvited."

"See, I told you I was a peculiar guy," he says. "But being here gives me such psychic rewards. I get pats on the back all the time from the guys. They tell me, 'I want to be like you when I'm eighty-five—a horny old man.' "

Yes, Nonas's horniness is a staple of his business, a comforting idiosyncrasy that, in its own small way, tells his bald customers, "You know what? It's going to be OK. You're still going to be bald. You're going to wear a toupee and you're going to get laid."

Which are, after all, the only words a man wants to hear.

That's the unstated deal, the Faustian bargain being offered by all the modern rug men. Every pamphlet, every newsletter, every in-fomercial, every "Best Little Hair House" ad campaign for hair-pieces carries with it an explicit sexual promise. Whether it's the video of that hairpiece wearer coming out of the pool (yes, you can wear it in the pool!) to join a hot babe on a lounge chair or a photo of a quiet, candlelit dinner à deux, bald men are given a chance to see themselves for what they are: normal, vibrant, sexual beings who just need a little covering up to achieve their goals.

Masculinity in all its forms—sex, athleticism, boozy cama-raderie—is inseparable from the pitch. A typical Hair Club for Men infomercial opens with shots of bald men reluctantly, almost tragi-cally, combing through their hair. One will look at the camera with big bloodhound eyes and say, "This can't be happening to me."

The viewer, most likely watching the infomercial in a weak mo-ment in the middle of the night, immediately identifies. He has said it to himself a million times: "How could I—a virile, successful, happy man—be losing my hair?" And, more important, "How can I *be* a virile, successful, happy man if I *keep* losing my hair?"

In case he needs a reminder, the weak, middle-of-the-night viewer is chided into action by the infomercial. "In our youthful oriented so-ciety," the fake newswoman/hostess says at one point, "it's tough for anyone to accept hair loss at any age. . . . We idolize youth."

But of course there is a solution. One client, Darryl, is shown in "before" photos as just starting to go bald. He says he tried Rogaine and saw no improvement and didn't consider a hair transplant. So he got a piece.

"I've never felt this good," he says, although his "after" photo is arguably a little too hairy. And then the clincher: "My wife likes the way I look and she likes the way she feels . . . When I come out of the shower, it's like I was a teenager again."

The way she *feels*? Coming out of the *shower*? A *teenager* again? Remind me again what is being sold here.

Toward the end of the infomercial, the fake newswoman/hostess gets caught up in the sexual energy, too, actually running her hands through Darryl's newfound hair, repeatedly moaning, "Umm, it feels so good!"

It's unabashed, certainly. But without sex, how are you going to sell a man a glued-on mat of someone else's hair?

Russo doesn't need to sell sex because by the time a man enters Top Priority to buy a toupee, the customer has already made his bargain. But that doesn't absolve Russo from the critical cheerleading role.

"Let's face it, when you're twenty-seven and you're bald, you just don't look as good," Russo says, recalling the age when he lost his hair. "I tell them not to think of a hairpiece as anything but a grooming aid. Or as part of their clothes."

Russo takes off his hairpiece every night—"Unless I get lucky!" he tells clients (a purposeful reminder of the sexy seventies). I ask him to take it off so I can see the full impact it makes on a man of his fifty years. He tugs at the three places where there's double-stick tape and removes it cleanly. Suddenly he ages twenty-five years, going from a guy who could pass for a Duran Duran frontman into a guy who looks like Paul Simon did during those unfortunate years when he sported his own horseshoe-style bald head.

He quickly puts the piece back on his head and straightens himself in the mirror.

"With my hair on, I look at myself and say, 'Not bad!' I look forty and have my old confidence back."

Russo's own experience with his hair recalls a segment done by a TV newsmagazine a few years back in which a bald man was sent into a crowded, singles-filled bar but comes out empty-handed. When he is sent in later with a good-looking hairpiece, he comes out with two phone numbers.

"Some day I might be able to just stop wearing it, maybe when I retire down to the Florida Keys and just sit around and fish, but not now," Russo says. "I'm still single and you need the hair to get the girl."

Like Nonas with his frat-house camaraderie or Russo, whose own toupee subtly reminds his customers that "we're all just fifty-year-old men trying to look like forty-year-old men so we can get laid," Sperling has fashioned his own club, the Hair Club for Men. Some of the principles are the same—central among them is make men feel like men again—but Sperling has done his old rival Nonas, whom he affectionately calls "Nonuts," one better.

Thanks only to Sperling—and, yes, his famous line, "I'm not only the Hair Club for Men president, but I'm also a client"—Hair Club for Men is inarguably the most widely known vendor of hairpieces. But beyond that, Hair Club has done more to popularize and mainstream the hairpiece than any single organization.

This has mainly been accomplished by never calling the product a toupee. In fact, never calling it anything but "hair."

Until recently Hair Club for Men did not even tell its prospective customers what, in fact, they were considering. There was frequent talk of "having your hair back" or of their exclusive "method of hair enhancement that is internationally recognized as state-of-the-art," but brochures only went as far as saying "Hair Club for Men offers a safe, natural looking, full head of hair for the man who cares about his appearance."

Full head of hair? Whose hair? You were not told until much farther along in the sales process.

"Their key strategy was never mentioning what they did exactly," says Spencer Kobren, a consumer advocate for bald men and author of *The Bald Truth,* an invaluable guide to the baldness industry. At that time, "Sy Sperling made it seem that Hair Club was the kind of club that, when joined, hair would magically appear on your head."

But Sperling has done much more than sell hairpieces. Like Nonas, Sperling has spent the last thirty years marketing the hairpiece as a cultural icon worthy of a place in mainstream society rather than a rug that men purchase with a whisper and a glance over their shoulders and stuff in a brown paper bag.

Sperling has always been a staple on late-night television—and not just through his infomercials. The specter of Sperling casts a long shadow over the advertising industry. His famous line about being the president and client has been appropriated into dozens of other ad campaigns for products as diverse as the NYNEX Yellow Pages to M&Ms and is as much a part of the culture as "Show me the money!" "Here's looking at you, kid," or "Where's the beef?"

But beyond that, on any given night—sometimes for no reason except the humor that comes from incongruity—you might find Sy Sperling chatting with David Letterman, trading lines with Lorne Michaels on *Saturday Night Live,* doing a fake infomercial for "The Hair Club for Wolfmen" or spending an hour in a box with Nipsey Russell for a hilarious bit of existential comedy on the *Conan O'Brien Show.*

"Can I show you my grandkids?" the box-imprisoned Sperling asks his fellow prisoner Russell, handing over his wallet.

Russell, expecting photos, is surprised. "These are credit cards, man," he says.

"Don't you judge me!" Sperling replies, becoming suddenly, inexplicably livid. "Don't you *dare* judge me!"

And who could forget Sperling's on-scene reporting for Jay Leno from the trial of O. J. Simpson? "Jay," Sperling said, a fake courtroom backdrop behind him, "both sides are losing . . . their hair!" And later, "Jay, there's no way to suppress the evidence . . . of Robert Shapiro's male pattern baldness!"

Meeting Sperling at the Hair Club offices in, appropriately, Boca

Raton, Florida, I ask him about those scores of comedy spots to see whether Sperling's self-effacing strategy is the product of design or coincidence.

"It shows I don't take myself too seriously," says Sperling. "Not many people would get in a box with Nipsey Russell and just say stupid things."

I tell him that he's underestimating himself, that the cameos and the self-mockery have done far more than turn Sperling into the best-known, best-loved hairpiece salesmen in America and direct men to go through the door of the local Hair Club office, but, more important, have helped create a world in which wearing a toupee is just not a big deal anymore.

"Yeah, I guess you're right," Sperling says. "The goal is to show people that no one is perfect. Maybe you need hair. Maybe that guy needs caps on his teeth. Someone else needs some cosmetics to cover up a scar. What's the big deal?"

Unlike Nonas, who was a successful ad man before he got his first toupee, Sperling, like many men of his generation, recalls feeling disenfranchised by his loss of hair. He had been recently divorced, and his baldness had made him feel like a 1950s square peg in the round hole of the swinging sixties, an opera-loving Giuliani in hip-hop New York.

But back then there were few options. Hair transplants were becoming more popular, but Sperling wisely rejected them as "too primitive." And toupees also left him less than impressed. "They were like dentures to me," he says.

And then he met Walter Tucciarone.

The hair weave concept—which called for strands of hair to be woven through combed-over rows of your own hair—had been around for a few years, but Tucciarone, whose family had been in the hair business since the turn of the century (and still is, thanks to Walter's son, Billy, and grandson, Billy Junior, who are both human hair importers in the Bronx), had just started mass-marketing it.

"Every piece of hair that goes into your head has a piece of Walter Tucciarone's brain in it," Walter would say.

That sounded good enough for Sperling, a pool salesman at the time. He wanted to go into business with Tucciarone, so he bought one of the weaves from the old man, a show of faith and the first time Sperling would serve as his own guinea pig.

"He finished the job and it looked absolutely great," Sperling recalls. "He tells me to treat it like my own hair, so I'm driving home and I'm singing and laughing and I'm happier than I've been in years. I can't wait to get home to take a shower and see how it looks."

As it turned out, Sperling could have waited. Rather than being like his own hair, the weave came out of the shower looking like a dead rat.

"It had curled up into a ball," Sperling says. "It was horrible. I spent the next three hours, no exaggeration, in front of the mirror trying to get it to look right again. My eyes were bloodshot. It was the greatest high in my life to the lowest low in the same day. My whole dream came crashing down."

Sperling's brother-in-law came over that night and ended up cutting the entire weave off Sperling's head. "I just said, 'Get this fucking thing off my head!' "

Naturally, a visit was paid to the Tucciarone shop.

"I said to Walter, 'This is a fraud. I don't want to go into business with you. You're a fucking liar.' "

But, as Sperling describes it, his "desperate need" calmed him down and Tucciarone was able to get out of the jam by offering Sperling something even better than a weave: a Tucci Original!

By any other name, a Tucci Original was a toupee, pure and simple: a thin mesh with hair sewn into it that would be tied into a man's side locks. When Sperling returned two days later to see the finished product, he was a little less than enthusiastic.

"Walter," he said, "that looks like a toupee you're weaving into my hair. I'm not going to wear a toupee."

So Tucciarone worked his magic. In his strong Italian accent, he told Sperling the lesson that would stay with him for the rest of his life: "You never say 'toupee.' Toupee cost two hondred! A Tucci Original cost *seven* hondred!"

Despite his prejudice against toupees, Sperling realized the Tucci Original was just what he needed. It looked good. He could shower with it. He could swim with it. And it didn't have to come off at night. So Tucciarone and Sperling were back in business, the great hair man manufacturing the product and the ex–pool salesman marketing it.

"We took a product that was selling for two hundred dollars and had a bad image and turned it into something we sold for seven hundred and had a good image," Sperling says. "Walter would get his two hundred and I would get my five hundred."

If that doesn't sound fair to you, you can imagine how Walter Tucciarone felt. Here was a guy who created the Tucci Original only to see his work be remarketed by Sperling, who took the better part of the profits.

"He saw how many we were selling, so he said, 'This isn't going to work. I should be making five hondred dollars and you should be making two hondred. Get out of here!' "

That might have been the end of Sy Sperling's career as a rug man except for one thing: He still had the Tucci Original.

"We showed it to another hairpiece maker and, suffice it to say, it wasn't an 'Original' for very long," Sperling says, laughing.

On his own, Sperling started Hair Recreations, which was the precursor to the modern Hair Club for Men. And even then he was also a client.

"I attribute much of my success in life to my personal experience with the hair," he says. "It did a lot to my self-esteem. I was thirty pounds heavier, yet I started taking care of myself. I bought new clothing. I was more positive in everything I did. When you believe in the product so strongly, it makes it easier to sell it. I'd show clients pictures and say, 'This is what I looked like and this is what I look like now.' I mean, it's true. I'm not only the president, I'm also a client, so I have a tremendous empathy with anyone who loses his hair. I truly understand what he's going through."

Today Hair Club is a $250-million business with eighty franchises throughout the country. And Sperling is still its number one-client—although, truth be told, the product doesn't look as good on him as it does on other men because Sperling's thin side hair looks ill-matched to the fuller hairpiece. (Employees whisper that they wish he'd move to a slightly thinner model that's more appropriate to his age of fifty-nine.)

What's more, Sperling is about to reinvent his company, moving it from only hairpieces to more of a full-service hair-loss superstore. He's already selling cover-up products, such as Toppik and COU-VRe made by Spencer Forrest, and now his research and development team is even investigating whether to include hair transplants under the Hair Club for Men umbrella.

"We're not going to get swept under the rug," said Sperling's spokesman Mike Smith (yes, he really said "swept under the rug"), explaining why Hair Club monitors such things as Dr. Angela Christiano's gene research at Columbia University and hair transplant conferences.

All this talk of the future has even led to Sperling being much more up-front about just what his product is. For the first time Hair Club brochures now include a detailed description of the product. It's all there: a description of the glue (sorry, "a very special polymer we call Polyfuse"), details about the base of the hairpiece ("the matrix is virtually invisible") and how the hair is fastened.

"It's far more graphic than it was," Sperling says, adding that Hair Club's less-than-forthcoming approach was necessary when the product—"a toupee?!"—was so widely ridiculed.

"When you're selling a product, you're selling the sizzle, not the steak," Sperling explains. "We were selling the fact that the guy would sit in the chair and look great two hours later. That's the sizzle. Think about hair transplant doctors. They sell the sizzle—you're going to look better—but not the steak. If they showed you the bloody photos, you'd never agree to the procedure. That's why I never referred to it as a toupee or a hairpiece. That's why Tucciarone sold it to me as a Tucci Original."

But when Sperling shows me a sample of the Hair Club hairpiece—which is made in his own factory in China—I can't help noticing that it looks suspiciously like one of Nonas's Virtual Reality models, also made in the Far East.

"It's not a toupee!" Sperling insists. "If you start calling it a toupee, the consumer will just lump it in with all the toupees and then all the work we've done perfecting it for twenty-five years is worthless. We've taken the word 'toupee' out of the language. 'Toupee' is a word that you think of when you watch the Three Stooges and someone knocks Moe's hair off of his head with a violin bow."

Even Nonas has begrudging respect for the man who took the hairpiece to new heights.

"I think Hair Club makes a fine product," Nonas says. "I just wish Sy would call it what it is: a toupee!"

*Chapter 5*

—

# THE BIG COVER-UP: FROM
# "HAIR-IN-A-CAN" TO SHEEP
# PROTEIN IN A BOTTLE

"Does not nature itself teach you that for a man to wear long hair is
degrading to him, but if a woman wears long hair it is her pride?"
—PAUL, in his first letter to the Corinthians

I recently had the pleasure of walking several blocks behind an
aging Borscht Belt comedian of substantial renown. As he walked
through Times Square—presumably toward the theater where he
had been performing—the crowds in front of us gawked and whis-
pered his name as he passed.

Oh, but if they only could've seen what I was seeing.

Walking just a pace or two behind afforded me a view of the dark
underbelly of celebrity that few get to see and none would know-
ingly *choose* to see. That he was balding did not surprise me. After
all, this man was well into his seventies. But as we walked, I found
that I simply could not take my eyes off his bald spot. There was
something altogether not right about it, something defiant of nature
and the aging process yet simplistic and monochromatic.

He was using spray-on hair!

It was unmistakable. He had taken what little hair he had,
combed it over his bald spot and subjected it to a barrage of aerosol
spraying that left each hair matted down and thickened with a coat

of cosmetic gunk. Yes, it matched the color of his scalp to the color of his hair, yet it succeeded only in making the bald spot that much more obvious.

Instead of retaining its natural strand configuration, his hairs had become clump-bearing filaments trapped against his head like bugs in a roach motel.

I could never look at celebrities the same way again. I was onto them now.

Just as my strolling comedian is not the first bald man to seek comfort in the cosmetics aisles of his local drugstore, I'm clearly not the first person to remark upon the absurdity of covering up one's bald spot with the cosmetic equivalent of paint.

Martial, the first-century Roman satirist, focused his rapier wit on the Romans' version of the much-maligned spray-on hair. Before there were such things as statically charged keratin fibers or aerosolized cosmetics (more on them later), bald Romans would think nothing of concealing their bald patches with rudimentary paint.

The results didn't look much better than what I saw during my after-work stroll through Times Square, if Martial is to be believed.

"You fob us off with fictitious hair," he wrote in a satire of upper-class Romans. "Your dirty bald scalp is covered with locks represented in paint. You have no occasion for a barber for your head; you may shave yourself much better, Phoebus, with a sponge."

Today, there are no products as widely ridiculed as male baldness cosmetics. Despite the fact that women have been covering up their slight imperfections for centuries with nary a snide remark, cover-up products for male pattern baldness provide punch lines for late-night talk shows, subplots in sitcoms and plenty of cocktail party ribbing.

"Whenever I meet people at a party and tell them what I do, they say, 'Oh, you make shoe polish for the head,' " said Mark Kress, president of Spencer Forrest, the leading maker of cover-up products [http://www.toppik.com]. "There have been so many jokes that the entire concept has become trivialized, but the people who buy it keep buying it because they know it works."

"Shoe polish for the head" is one way to put it. Watching an old infomercial for a Ronco spray-on product called "Great Looking Hair Formula 9," you can't help but be struck by the sense that you are either witnessing one of the greatest moments in intentional, postmodern self-parody or the lowest moment in the history of commerce.

"My God, look how big Paco's bald spot is!" shrieks the infomercial's perky hostess. "What can you do for him, Ron?"

She is talking to Ron Popeil, the mastermind behind GLH9, as well as such revolutionary "as-seen-on-TV" products as the Popeil Pocket Fisherman, the Smokeless Ashtray, Mr. Microphone and his new home rotisserie grill [http://www.ronco.com]. On the infomercial, Popeil grabs a can of GLH9 and releases such a torrent of the product onto Paco's head that you can see wisps of smoke flying everywhere. When he's done spraying, with the right camera work, it can look like a reasonable facsimile of a very average makeup job.

With the wrong lighting, though, it can look like the head of an old comedian walking through Times Square.

Or, as Pulitzer Prize–winning humor columnist Dave Barry once put it, it can look like a head that "has been dipped in roofing tar" or a head that "looked as though a professional baseball team had used [it] to groom the infield." (Barry also criticized the $9.95 for shipping and handling, saying that the vast majority of the money goes to "the extra salary they have to pay the operators for not laughing directly into the phone" when you order the product.)

But there must be something to baldness cosmetics—something the hair-covered mockers don't understand—or else Mark Kress wouldn't be driving a $70,000 Porsche Carrera, now would he?

Kress's car is just one indication that his Spencer Forrest, Inc.— which now sells Toppik shake-on hair fibers and Fullmore spray-on coverage in addition to its original cosmetic cream, COUVRe—is doing well.

Another is that picture behind his desk of him beaming and shaking hands with President Clinton and Vice President Gore at a 1999 Entrepreneur of the Year award ceremony.

Another is his own head—the final laboratory for so many Spencer Forrest developments over the years. In fact, he swears he sprinkled Toppik fibers onto his bald spot just before meeting the president.

Like so many in the bald industrial complex today, Mark Kress did not go looking for baldness, baldness found him. He was thirty-five years old when he noticed the telltale thinning and the lemon-shaped flesh yarmulke that had developed on the crown of his head.

"I was single and in my thirties and I didn't like what I saw," said the fifty-five-year-old Kress, whom I met in the Westport, Connecticut, house that serves as his office and distribution point. (He picked me up at the train in the Porsche, by the way, and as we buzzed through some of the country's richest real estate, I couldn't suppress the feeling that there is, indeed, a parallel world of wealth and leisure of which I know, approximately, nothing.)

Kress, who today looks like a middle-aged Wolfman Jack [http://www.wolfmanjack.org/picgal.htm], tried hair transplants, starting with large plug grafts back in 1979, and has since had four transplants, each taking advantage of the field's increasing proficiency to the point where now, a few months after his most recent transplant, his hair looks great.

But it was that first transplant that led him to the "discovery" that would change his life, if not the lives of thousands of balding men and women and the comedians who mock them. It wasn't that he didn't like the transplant (men simply didn't know better then), but he found that once he'd undergone a cosmetic procedure, he could never look in the mirror the same way again.

You hear this a lot from surgeons who perform face-lifts, liposuction or other cosmetic operations; the minute the patient removes the gauze, he becomes obsessed with every tiny crease, every added pound or, in the case of hair transplant patients, every gap between two grafts.

"When I had the transplant, I found myself staring at my hair all the time," said Kress. "It only made me *more* conscious. So while I was recovering from the plugs and waiting for the hair to grow in, I was looking for a way to cover my baldness."

At the time, Kress said, the main cover-up-type product on the market was called Top Coverage—it's the classic "shoe polish" that men think of when they hear the term "hair-in-a-can."

Kress used it but was dissatisfied. The product adhered so strongly to the scalp, he said, that when he'd remove it at night, he'd be forced to remove some of his precious few hairs with it.

Fortunately for Kress, he had an entrepreneur's spirit, even if it was trapped in the body of a sales manager for a Los Angeles TV station.

"I was always interested in developing my own products, even though my background is in advertising and marketing," he said. "But when my personal needs combined with my desire to develop a product, everything started clicking."

With the help of a cosmetics expert, Kress developed the COU-VRe cream—which is a sesame oil emulsion that looks like cake frosting but goes on like women's makeup—while still working at the TV station. Although women had plenty of skin-care products and cosmetics, men simply did not.

"When I started COUVRe, there was no category," Kress said. "I had just assumed I'd flip through *GQ* or *Esquire* and see ads for these kinds of products because drugs and surgery still leave a need for them. But it wasn't out there, so I had to make it, which meant I wasn't only selling the product, but selling everyone on the idea that this was a legitimate cosmetic product for men."

A COUVRe commercial from this era captures Kress's frustration perfectly. In it, a dissatisfied bald man (hey, he's not just an actor, he's a dissatisfied bald man) looks at the camera and complains about all the failed methods for "curing" baldness.

"Now there's even spray paint!" he says with righteous outrage. "Hey, this isn't a piece of furniture—it's my head!"

COUVRe started slowly but eventually took off. Meanwhile, so did Kress's career (a coincidence, perhaps?). Even while he was making and selling COUVRe, he became the vice president for marketing for a large, West Coast–based radio network and, later, president and owner of Joan Rivers Productions (which created such vital television programming as *Can We Shop?*).

He eventually sold the company back to Rivers in 1995 to work on hair products full-time. Now he could refine his product.

The result is Toppik, which, unlike other baldness cover-ups, is neither a cosmetic nor an aerosol.

It's chopped-up sheep hair.

No, really, the most significant development in covering up male pattern baldness consists of keratinized fragments from the hair of merino wool sheep. The fibers are chopped into microscopic pieces, dyed and infused with a negative static charge so that they stick to your hair.

As ideas go, this isn't the most ingenious. For years, a backstage Hollywood secret of covering an actor's bald spot was to take some of the actor's extra hair, chop it finely with a razor blade (in the manner, say, of another Hollywood secret) and glue it artfully along the actor's receding hairline.

But Kress took it one step further by using sheep hair, which turns out to work best. Kress had tried powder and then synthetic fibers, but they didn't work because they won't hold a charge—and static cling is the secret of Toppik.

"It was a trial-and-error process," Kress said about the making of Toppik. "I had a consultant from the wool industry who did a lot of detective work. We found it works best on men with some peach fuzz up there. Through it all, the laboratory was my head."

To demonstrate its effectiveness to me, Kress prepared that laboratory for another experiment. First, he showed me his Gore-like bald patch, which is surrounded by just enough natural hair so that the Toppik will have a place to which to cling.

Kress then took a vial of the Toppik out of his top drawer (convenient, isn't it?) and tapped out the fibers onto his head as if he were shaking salt onto a roasted chicken. When he felt he'd released enough of the fibers, he patted his hair into place, allowing the bits of merino wool to settle and cling to different spots along the hair shafts around the bald spot and onto the scalp itself.

The result was hair that looked thicker without the gummy, caked-on look of so many other products. And because it's powder-like, any extra that fell onto clothes was simply brushed away. If you'd put a patch of Kress's treated head under a microscope, instead of seeing thin strands of hair that resemble bare autumn trees, you'd see the bounty of summer: hair that seems to sprout in every direction (even though all the "branches" are merely pieces of dyed sheep hair that are forced by the laws of electrophysics to stick to your hair).

It will stay on until you shampoo it off. And, more important for the Porsche-owning Kress, you can drive with the top down.

"I do use it, but only when I care about my appearance, like at a social function," Kress said. "That's why I had it on that day with the president." (Can anyone really blame him? I mean, if you're at the White House to celebrate your entrepreneurial talents, it never hurts to be using the fruits of your labor when you meet the president of the United States—especially when his vice president is so obviously, umm, sympathetic to the plight of bald men.)

Kress now claims that he has 300,000 customers—although he wouldn't give me actual sales figures because, let's face it, no one gives out sales figures of anything unless you're a government official with a subpoena. He actually claimed that if he told me how much business he does, other entrepreneurs would want a piece of Kress's sheep-hair-covered pie.

Glen Prytula would say he already *has* a piece. And Prytula, owner of DermMatch, a Venice, Florida–based company that sells a powdered cover-up product called (you guessed it) DermMatch, feels that his product is even better than Toppik.

"People complain that you can't swim in Toppik or that it falls out," Prytula said. "When you're dealing with these types of products, that's unacceptable because people don't want to be embarrassed. But you can swim in DermMatch and it won't drip."

Prytula then recited for me the company slogan, which is his pride and joy: "DermMatch: Nothing looks better, stays on better, applies neater, is more healthful or costs less to use." (If that's the company *slogan,* I'd hate to see the employee handbook.) [http://www.dermatch.com]

"It's wordy, but it covers each of the five areas that people who have hair loss are concerned about," Prytula said.

Though Prytula and Kress are bitter competitors, in another world, at another time, they might have been close friends. Like Kress, Prytula is going bald. And like Kress, Prytula's less-than-satisfying experience with hair transplants got him interested in finding an alternative.

And like Kress, Prytula hated his hair loss.

"It was very traumatic," he said. "Through no fault of my own, people started losing respect in me, just because I was losing hair. Around that time, I took a course in college that showed that the first thing we notice about each other is hair. If bald people didn't get a negative reaction from other humans there would be no market for these products. But you hear the remarks and you say, 'I don't need this,' so you take care of it."

Prytula uses his own product—a hard-packed, dry cosmetic that you rub directly onto the scalp—to fill in the gaps between his old-style plug grafts. Like COUVRe, the DermMatch powder masks the nudity of the scalp while, like Toppik, it also makes each hair shaft appear thicker.

"It's not going to make Kojak look like Elvis—nothing can do that," said Prytula, mixing pop culture with pop music, the seventies with the fifties. "But every little bit helps. DermMatch looks great. No one says to me, 'Hey, you painted your head!' "

Then again, people may just be being nice. Intrigued by the myriad of cover-up products on the market today, I convened a panel of experts to serve as guinea pigs for what I believe to be the world's first-ever, full-scale male cover-up-product test.

And the participants are: Toppik, the sheep hair in a can; COUVRe, the makeup cream; Fullmore, which is Spencer Forrest's spray-on powder; DermMatch, the powered cosmetic whose name sounds like a personal ad for someone looking for a skin transplant; and Great Looking Hair Formula 9, the legendary "spray-on hair" made and marketed by the master salesman Ron Popeil.

Should anyone wish to re-create my experiment, understand that all surfaces (including the computer on which you are taking notes and that half bagel you were saving for later) should be fully covered before beginning. Both of the spray-on products—Fullmore and GLH9—and, to a lesser degree, Toppik fibers tend to get airborne. Once they do, they go all over the place. And I mean *all over the place*. Into flowerpots, onto windowsills and mirrors, and all over the countertops. And don't forget your own orifices! Without being too graphic, let me just tell you that the day after my test, every time I blew my nose, black fibers and gunk came out.

That said, let's meet our panel of experts. First, there's my friend Eric, a small-business owner from Brooklyn, New York [http://www.penguin-place.com]. Eric has the early stages of classic male pattern baldness, with hair receding from his temples and leaving a thinning frontal forelock. The hair on the back of his head, though, is still quite full. Eric recently stopped using Propecia after a year because he felt it wasn't giving him great results. Since abandoning the pill, though, his hair loss has accelerated like an eighteen-wheeler with brake failure.

Did he have a choice, really? At $2 per pill per day, using Propecia for thirty years would have set him back nearly $22,000. Even Rogaine would cost nearly $7,000 over that same period. Like many bald men, Eric decided to cut his losses, although he misses his hair.

Joining Eric is my friend Mark, an actor whose occupation makes him somewhat preoccupied with his looks. Unlike Eric, who has no hair in areas where it's receded, Mark has some coverage of the thinning areas of his crown and vertex. He is the perfect candidate for these products, their makers said.

Now, to the results.

We started with Toppik, the newest and most sophisticated of the products. Unlike the others, Toppik is actually fun to use (shaking sheep hair onto your friends' heads sure beats a day job). With every shake of the small, pocket-sized Toppik bottle, you can see bald spots disappearing, especially for a guy like Mark, whose bald patch has just enough peach fuzz to provide the perfect base.

When the dust had settled (literally), Mark found himself acting like those paid actors on infomercials, screaming "Oh my God!" around the house like someone had tapped him with a magic wand and he had regressed fifteen years to his hairy boyhood.

Even my wife, who regards it a crime to cover up what nature has doled out, was impressed.

Eric did not enjoy as much success with Toppik because the sheep hair needs some human hair to which to attach itself. On Eric's denuded patches, Toppik merely looked like someone had sprinkled copy machine toner onto his head, not a good look (even if you work for Xerox).

COUVRe was an unmitigated disaster for both men. The product, which is applied with a triangular makeup sponge, does not go on easily because your hair keeps getting in the way. The goal is to get the COUVRe to the scalp, but if you have too much hair, it never makes it, and instead clumps up.

For Mark, it looked like someone had taken a Magic Marker to his head. Eric looked at himself in the mirror and screamed, "It looks like I'm in a racially offensive minstrel show from the 1920s! Get this stuff off me!"

Fullmore, the third Spencer Forrest product, also did not seem as effective as Toppik. Both men found the spray bouncing off them and into the surrounding air (and, apparently, up my nose). No matter how much we used, the balding areas refused to be properly covered. And what *was* covered felt gritty and cakey.

I urged both testers to resist the temptation to see DermMatch as shoe polish for the head. It was difficult, at times, considering that DermMatch's hard-packed cosmetic powder is shipped in thin containers that look identical to shoe-polish discs. It's applied after first dampening it with moistened wands that resemble large Q-Tips and then rubbing it into the scalp.

So maybe it was inevitable that Mark and Eric would see DermMatch as little better than bootblack. "It really does look like shoe polish on my head," Mark said. "It looks like a dark arrow of electrical tape pointing directly at my bald spot," added Eric. Both men felt the product had the same limitations as COUVRe.

Now, before discussing what happened with GLH9, I need to make the following disclaimer: Ron Popeil, a man I have respected for many years, a man whose inventions are as much a part of every American home as a K-Tel eight-track (yes, *that* Ron Popeil), initially balked at sending me some of his "amazing hair product" out of fear that I would improperly apply it and then write negative things about it.

Ron, I can assure you: I would never do that (the former, that is; I can't make any promises about the latter).

"You have to hold it an inch from the head—but nobody knows what an inch is!" Popeil told me by phone from his California office.

He then proceeded to tell me a story about his one-man crusade to rescue his much-ridiculed product. It was back in the mid-1990s when a reporter from *USA Today* called Popeil to get a sample of his product for a story the paper was doing on, well, spray-on hair. Popeil refused, but offered to *bring* the reporter the sample, if Popeil himself could apply it to bald men at the paper's Virginia headquarters. The deal was struck.

"I was spraying all these people and everyone was satisfied," said Popeil. "Of course, it was on the front page and they gave me almost the whole page. And they said positive things about it."

I know what that's like. The last time I met Popeil face-to-face, back in 1995 when he was on a tour promoting his book *Salesman of the Century,* Popeil stripped down naked in front of me because I admitted I had never seen GLH9 in action.

Within seconds, he was spraying his head jet-black. "Isn't that amazing?" he said in his standard TV patter when he was done.

What is more amazing is the energy Popeil puts into everything he does. Since making the jump from selling his vegetable slicers on the state fair circuit to selling them on TV, Popeil has sold more than one billion Ronco products and turned his advertising come-ons into national catchphrases.

"*Now* how much would you pay? Wait, don't answer . . ." That was his.

"Slice an onion and the only tears you'll cry will be tears of joy." That was his, too.

"So sharp, you could cut a cow in half—and that's no bull!"

This guy could sell Snoop Doggy Dogg records to Joe Lieberman.

So naturally I promised to read all the GLH9 directions and watch the accompanying videotape, "GLH9 Cosmetic Hair Thickener Instructional Video With Styling Tips From Ron Popeil." On my word, Popeil sent me a can of spray-on hair. "Too many people enjoy this product for me to believe it won't work for you," he said.

Have those people call my friends Mark and Eric. The product, used as directed, did not work for them.

"I love his rotisserie grill, but this stuff is pasty and it comes off in your hands," said Mark. "And if you don't get the color matched perfectly, it looks like you dipped your head into a can of paint."

"From a distance, it looks plausible, but up close you can see what's going on here," Eric added. "It really is like a powdered version of black paint."

In the end, both men came to learn a valuable lesson about these products, and themselves.

"You know, when you're sitting there spraying your head with an aerosol can of powder, you have to stop and say to yourself, 'Why am I doing this?' " Mark said. "At some point, you have to say, 'Is baldness so bad?' "

You can say it all you want, but society will still say otherwise. It remains one of the great ironies of baldness that a condition experienced by more than half the male population is, nonetheless, a cause for ridicule, scorn and heartlessness.

"We live in a society where everyone always wants to look younger," said the sixty-something Popeil, who, with his thirty-something wife and his one-year-old child, is living proof that people tend to be more attracted to youth.

"Listen, a single guy doesn't want to end up with an old-looking woman, just like a young woman doesn't want to end up with an old-looking man. They want to go out and be around other attractive people. That's how society positions us. If a young lady sees a bald spot on me, she's going to think I'm too old."

At sixty-six, he is. No wonder he was wearing GLH9 when he met his wife.

"So I color my hair, what's the big deal?" Popeil asked. "I have a young wife and I don't want people saying to me, as has happened in the past, 'Your daughter is nice.' She's not my daughter, she's my *wife*! Everyone is vain to some degree. Some more than others. And I'm a vain individual. I care how I look."

As passionately as Popeil talks about his GLH9 cover-up, it pales in comparison to the ardor he has for his latest creation, the in-home rotisserie grill. In fact, just trying to keep Popeil on the topic of baldness was next to impossible. Popeil is no shyster, no snake-oil salesman. He believes in his products and they work for many people. But to hear him talking about "revolutionary" kitchen products one second and his "amazing" baldness cover-up the next made me feel that his commitment to helping bald men is more commercial than spiritual. Are the heads of bald men just raw chickens to be grilled or onions to be sliced? Apparently so.

"I sold forty thousand rotisseries this week! This week!" he said when I asked my very first question about GLH9.

Popeil created GLH9 almost a decade ago, and you can just hear the air wheezing out of that balloon. The infomercial the company sent me was at least five years old, and even Popeil admitted that he's lost interest in GLH9. This is a man who must constantly be in motion—but forward only, toward the invention and marketing of new products.

"GLH was a phenomenal product—it still is—but the rotisserie is the greatest for me," he said. "I ran into Larry King—Larry King!—the other day and he says to me, 'That fucking rotisserie! It's awesome!' Larry King!"

But did he say anything about GLH9?

"Nah, I didn't ask."

*Chapter 6*

—

# A MASTER'S TROUBLED LEGACY:
# THE TRANSPLANTATION OF HAIR

"Good looks can open doors, but good hair blows them off the hinges."
—SAM MALONE, the bartender played by Ted Danson on *Cheers*

She wants to know if I can handle the blood.

I am in the office of New York hair transplantation surgeon Michael Reed awaiting the arrival of a bald man who doesn't want to be. As Ronda Olinsky, one of Reed's assistants, lays out a series of instruments that gets increasingly terrifying—scissors, tweezers, a four-toothed curled retractor, long-needled syringes filled with anesthesia and, last, a menacing scalpel—she is concerned that no one has prepared me for the operation I am about to watch.

"Are you going to be OK with all the blood?" Olinsky asks, making it sound as if I am about to witness a Civil War–era double amputation after eating a full breakfast. "There's one gory part. Didn't they tell you?"

Olinsky is referring to the removal of the patient's "donor site," the excruciating but surprisingly quick initial stage of the three-hour procedure that involves slicing off a thick band of flesh from the back of the patient's head, cutting it free with surgical scissors and then cauterizing the bleeders until the operating theater smells of burnt flesh.

"It can overwhelm some people," Olinsky concludes as she finishes setting up the room.

I'm about to tell her that maybe I should be taking the same 2-milligram dose of Lorazepam—a sedative—that Reed's patient has just been given in the waiting room. But before I can get the joke out, the patient is brought in and I get my first chance to look at the head of a man who believes that his happiness depends upon a $5,000 operation to counteract millennia of human evolution.

Objectively speaking, Tony is not bald. When Reed combs Tony's hair forward into a "Caesar" for the preop photos, it is clear that Tony's hair loss would be noticeable only to close friends or casting agents.

But that's not the point of hair transplantation. People don't undergo the procedure—a physically uncomfortable, emotionally difficult and financially draining one—because of how strangers view them in the street. They get the procedure because of how they view themselves in the mirror. They look at themselves and see not the young adult they remember, but an old guy with no hair. Or worse, a frail, mortal version of themselves. *That can't possibly be me, could it?*

In cases of early balding like Tony's, some surgeons might not recommend a transplant—just dose him up with Propecia and Rogaine and see how he looks in a year. But Tony wants the operation and, more important, can pay for it, so it's ultimately his call.

"Tony has seventy percent of his hair left," Reed says. "You're not considered bald until you've lost fifty percent of your hair. But when he looks in the mirror, he sees a bald guy. So that's why he's here."

Reed is a respected hair transplant provider in several key ways. For one, he does all his own work, from the basic anesthetizing to the removal of the donor strip to the suturing of the wound to the punching of the recipient sites to the tedious and rote insertion of the hair grafts themselves—jobs that transplant mills and even many legitimate doctors sometimes delegate to subordinates even though it is illegal. Reed's Manhattan office is not a transplant factory, but a sober place of dermatologic medicine where no more than one transplant is done per day. Some practices cut up and replant a half dozen men in the same busy workday.

Reed selects the donor site by combing through the hair on the back of Tony's head. When he's satisfied, he shaves the hair, leaving only stubs that will ease the dissection process later. Throughout the process, there is very little doctor-patient interaction, something I noticed at other procedures I witnessed, no matter who was performing the operation. Medicine is not about personal contact between doctor and patient. In fact, it's probably about the opposite; if the doctor gets too chummy with the patient, it makes it harder to stick a scalpel into perfectly healthy flesh.

"First, do no harm" does not apply to cosmetic surgery.

Reed finally breaks the businesslike silence because there's something that he simply must point out: "You have a beautiful donor site," he tells Tony as he uses a blue Sharpie to mark off an area of his patient's head that will soon not be.

Tony doesn't know how to respond to the compliment, so he mutely lies facedown on the examination table, his face supported by a cushioned "doughnut," so that Reed can liberate the healthy hair follicles.

I will soon know if I can handle the blood. I'm not sure I can handle the anesthesia.

Anesthetizing a 15-centimeter swath across the back of a head requires far more than just one injection. Because the donor site is so long, Reed injects one spot, pushes the plunger a few centimeters, pulls out and repeats the process an inch to the right. When the vessel is empty, he hands it to a nurse, who gives him another full syringe, which he quickly empties. There's nothing dainty or polite about the process; Reed quickly slips the needle deep into Tony's subcutaneous fat, punches the plunger and then pulls out the needle just as rapidly, proceeding across Tony's head with a stick-and-move style that would be the envy of Mike Tyson. At once, Reed is a serial anesthetizer, a mob knife man, the Demon Numb-er of East Sixty-first Street.

Next, he repeats the rapid process with a longer-lasting anesthesia. By the time Reed is done, about 6 cc's of Xylocaine, the short-lasting local; about 12 cc's of marcaine, the longer-lasting knockout juice; and 30 to 60 cc's of simple saline solution (to stiffen the area for cutting) have been pumped into Tony's donor site, swelling it like a bloodworm engorged after a storm. But there's no risk of overdose, Reed says, because the donor strip will be gone long before the anesthetic has time to seep into Tony's system.

While Reed and his team put on rubber gloves, all the little injection holes start dripping blood, which runs into little rivers that meet in reservoirs behind Tony's ears. He can feel it, the sticky hot liquid running down his cheek, while the nurses talk about Barbra Streisand.

The blood is nothing compared with what happens next. Almost without effort, half of Reed's scalpel blade disappears into Tony's head and Reed begins cutting along his blue line, slicing in the downward direction in which the hair is growing. The cut is on an angle, and I can't help thinking that he's slicing Tony's scalp exactly the way one carves up a barbecued flank steak—across the grain and on the bias. He uses the same technique to cut along his bottom line until he has carved out a flattened ellipse.

But the piece is still attached to the bed of subcutaneous fat just below the dermal level. Picking up one corner with forceps, Reed uses scissors to free the donor area. The scissors make a noise that sounds far more like ripping than slicing—and, indeed, some doctors actually prefer ripping the strip directly out of the head rather than scissoring it. Within a few snips, though, the entire swath of Tony's skin is free, and Reed holds it up for everyone to inspect.

Stories about the donor site removal alone are enough to make many bald men reject the procedure. When he was coming to terms with his own baldness, *New York Times* sportswriter Richard Sandomir contemplated getting a transplant, but was turned off merely by watching this part of the operation. "Watching it is like the feeling you get when a ballplayer gets hit by a ball in his groin and he can't hold it in front of 50,000 people," he wrote in *Bald Like Me.* "What empathy you feel!"

My own emotions were closer to confusion. I could not help wondering why anyone would do this and why highly skilled surgeons like Reed would even bother. When I think of medicine, I think of lives saved, not follicles relocated to a safer neighborhood. You never saw George Clooney performing an emergency liposuction on *ER*.

But then again, you never see TV shows deal with the pain bald men feel when their hair recedes. That pain is real no matter how benign or trivial baldness is.

So what's wrong with a little follicular busing?

"Why not [operate], if the patient earnestly requests it and has an otherwise healthy personality?" asked University of Pennsylvania dermatology professor Albert Kligman.

With its stubby hairs on top and layer of bright yellow fat on the bottom, the donor strip looks like an animal pelt or, more specifically, the underside of the tail on a coonskin cap. If it seems strange, consider that this type of donor harvesting replaced "shotgun" harvesting, where surgeons would punch out large grafts from the back of the head, leaving gaps that healed unevenly and made it difficult to get more grafts for future operations. "Strip" harvesting became standard operating procedure in the 1970s and turned out to be the vital first step in the revolution toward increasingly smaller grafts.

Reed again admires Tony's "beautiful" donor site for just a second before returning to the matter at hand: his patient's open scalp.

Watching hair transplantation surgery shatters the comforting illusion that the body is one cohesive unit, a collection of parts all working together for a grand, noble purpose rather than a series of attached, but wholly independent, pieces.

Sure, there's blood issuing from a few spots on Tony's head, but for the most part, it looks as though the patient could just get up off the table and walk out into Midtown Manhattan without any problems except possible infection. A half-inch-wide, one-eighth-inch-deep segment of his head might be missing, but the rest of his body goes about its business like a plane on autopilot.

Reed grabs the infrared coagulator, an implausibly sci-fi-looking device that cauterizes blood vessels. Despite its high-tech appearance, the device is decidedly medieval; Reed holds the working end against each bleeder and pulls the trigger. The device sizzles and a burnt smell fills the room. If Tony wasn't anesthetized, someone would have to give him a bullet to bite.

The bleeding stopped, Reed checks the patient's head before closing. "You have such a succulent scalp," he says. It's easy work, so as he stitches Tony's head together with standard surgical double knots, Reed chats about the Alamo ("It's in San Antonio, not Houston!"), margaritas and medical supplies he needs to order.

And that's that. The "gory part" has passed with no fainting reporters, no lost lunches. Meanwhile, in another room, Reed's technicians are already hard at work on the donor site, dissecting it under microscopes into one-, two- and three-hair "single follicular units" that will later be implanted into small holes punched into Tony's head.

Their relentless dissection points up the inherent contradiction of hair transplantation. As a medical procedure, it is at once eminently logical and preposterously ridiculous to take healthy hair from one part of the scalp and transplant it into a part of the scalp that is barren.

Transplants no longer have the power to shock. Nowadays, scientists are transplanting all manner of human tissue. Where once the public thought of transplants as cutting-edge medicine or warily questioned the ethics of such new technology, transplant surgery now barely elicits news coverage.

We even got bored with the transplanted hand.

And, after all, what's the big deal about a transplant? If a man's kidneys fail him, should he not receive a working one from someone else? If skin is needed to cover a burned area, should it not be taken from another area of the body where it is superfluous?

Of course, but when the topic is hair, transplants are viewed with suspicion. Even the most accomplished and successful hair transplant surgeons admit that the transfer of hair follicles from the hairy back of one's head to the balding top has a quality of the absurd. As one skeptical dermatologist pointed out, the procedure doesn't create new follicles, it merely moves the healthy ones around.

Robbing Peter to pay Paul is a principle that governs many medical procedures. But in the case of hair, Paul is being paid so he can squander the money on expensive cosmetic surgery.

That is not to disparage men's motivations for getting a hair transplant. There's plenty of evidence that bald men often suffer profound effects of their hair loss. They feel older. They feel unattractive. They can't even get elected to higher office. Many withdraw from social settings, gain weight or lose self-esteem, beginning a cycle that becomes a self-fulfilling prophecy.

Of course, not every bald man is affected by his hair loss.

"I don't *suffer* from baldness," Reed says. Indeed, his hair is thinning badly and old photos on his desk and walls show how quickly he has gone from thinning to balding to bald—but, he claims, without the psychological toll other men face.

"I was eighteen when I started losing my hair and it was very traumatic," says Reed, one of dozens of hair transplant surgeons who are themselves bald. "But I'm a reasonably content guy and it doesn't bother me enough to go through a surgical procedure. Maybe I'd consider it if I was a fifty-year-old guy cruising the bars looking for women, which is a pathetic enough thing to begin with."

Robert Bernstein of the New Hair Institute is in Reed's camp. Bernstein has so little gray hair remaining on either side of his head that he resembles a lightbulb whose screw end has been dusted ever so lightly in flour.

Yet he is unbowed.

"For me, hair loss is no big deal," he says. "My father was bald and maybe it doesn't bother me because I had a great relationship with him."

And Bernstein, whom many feel is the conscience of the hair transplantation business, says he can see through the "Madison Avenue bullshit" that drives bald men crazy.

"Madison Avenue goes out and tells bald men that they don't look good, just like they tell women that they have to wear high heels or that men need to wear a thin tie this year, a wide tie next year and a shiny tie the year after that. Madison Avenue is all about creating dissatisfaction. *That's* the absurdity of hair transplants. It's absurd that our society places so much value on *hair.*"

Besides, when he was growing up, he had a horrible case of scoliosis, which required painful back surgery. The experience left him more philosophical about his hair loss. "Compared to the back pain, it was kind of trivial. I mean, so many people in this country lead such charmed lives. I can bet you that Chinese peasants aren't sitting around worrying about their hair loss."

On the other end of the spectrum is Dr. Gary Hitzig [http://www.877hairusa.com]. Like many hair transplant surgeons, Hitzig got into the business after battling his own baldness—and losing.

"When I lost my hair, I felt old, which is something a single guy in his twenties doesn't want to feel," said Hitzig, who has done about thirty thousand hair transplants in a long, checkered career (he's currently facing some malpractice suits from several dozen seriously dissatisfied patients; Hitzig stands by his work in all of these cases).

On the day that I visited Hitzig in his Manhattan office, he had just completed a 650-graft job—a $5,000 procedure—on a twenty-three-year-old whose hair had only begun thinning. Bernstein has said that he won't operate on men that young or who need so few grafts, yet Hitzig fully empathizes with the feelings of inadequacy men feel when their hair starts showing up at the bottom of the drain.

"Is a car expensive?" he says when I mutter that $5,000 is a lot to pay for hair. "This is investing in yourself. If you can make yourself look younger, you'll do better in life. Look at it this way—most CEOs have hair."

This isn't just the standard pitch of the hair transplanter. In fact, Hitzig is not just a hair transplant surgeon, he's also a hair transplant patient, a former toupee wearer, a snake-oil victim and a one-man pharmaceutical laboratory—all in his own historic quest to create the kind of mane he now promises his customers.

He got his first hair transplant—he's had nearly a half-dozen subsequent procedures—after being involved in an incident that, like the best slapstick, is only funny because it didn't happen to you.

One night while he was out on a date, a gust of wind blew Hitzig's toupee from his head and sent it hurtling down the sidewalk directly into the path of a woman carrying two grocery bags. When the flying hair collided with the terrified woman, she dropped the groceries, sending eggs and vegetables rolling all over the street.

"I just ran away, I was so embarrassed," Hitzig said. "I left the toupee right there and I never saw the girl again."

Eventually, he turned to transplants and, although unsatisfied by early, "pluggy" procedures, he's much happier with the recent ones done by his medical partner, John Schwinning. (Schwinning, by the way, is no longer licensed in New York State to perform anything other than hair transplants, a ruling by the New York State Health Department that he did not challenge because, he says, he wanted to devote himself fully to transplants anyway. It must be said that Schwinning is doing something right; the work he did on Hitzig is a gorgeous calling card and worthy of an "after" photo.)

The plug grafts that dissatisfied Hitzig when he was a patient were the same type of grafts that he transplanted in his own customers until fairly recently. The story of how plug grafts were invented—and how the medical community embraced them for far longer than it should have—is a classic example of how good money can make for bad medicine in cosmetic surgery, a field that sometimes has the hard-sell salesmanship of aluminum siding rather than the exhaustive rigor of science.

"It's not only the money, although that's a large part of it," said Emmanuel Marritt, a Colorado hair transplant surgeon who abandoned the business in 1999 after twenty years because he no longer felt he was doing good work.

That type of self-awareness is almost unheard of in hair transplantation. "There's a lot of inertia that most doctors feel when they've been doing a technique for a long time and think they're doing it well," Marritt added. "You get status in the business and if a newer, better technique comes along, there's a reluctance to suddenly admit that all the journal articles you wrote are suddenly obsolete."

Not to mention, Marritt said, having to reprint all your four-color brochures.

"If a new procedure comes around, most doctors don't even tell their patients about it," said Marritt, whose thoughts on the sleazy side of the transplant business will be presented in a sure-to-be-controversial book, *The Hair Replacement Revolution* (to be published in fall 2001 by Square One Publishing).

"It's modeled on Dickens's *A Tale of Two Cities*," he said, only slightly kidding. "In hair transplantation today, these are the best of times and the worst of times."

Hair transplantation as we know it was "invented" in 1952 by New York dermatologist Norman Orentreich almost entirely as an academic exercise. Orentreich had spent years combating various skin diseases, many of which caused hair loss, and was finally so frustrated (or is the better word "inspired"?) that he devised a simple experiment: He would punch out four plugs from a few dozen bald men—two from a part of the scalp where hair did not grow, two more from a part of the scalp where it did—replant them and see which ones grew and which ones did not.

Despite James Hamilton's research showing that hair loss was triggered by male sex hormones coursing through the arteries and attacking hair follicles that had a genetic predisposition toward baldness, many still believed that baldness was caused by poor blood flow to some regions of the scalp.

Orentreich [http://www.orentreich.com] was not the first man of medicine to move hair from one part of the head to another. It was first proposed in 1822 by a doctoral student in Germany named J. Dieffenbach, who experimented with transplanting hairs on a variety of animals.

Hair transplantation, however, did not take off until the 1930s in Japan, where doctors had succeeded in transplanting tiny amounts of hair to replace the eyebrows of victims of leprosy or burn. By World War II, the Japanese were far ahead of American hair doctors and would have surely succeeded in "inventing" the modern hair transplant were it not for World War II.

History tells us that hair was not a top priority for Japanese scientists during those years.

Knowing what Hamilton found, Orentreich accurately predicted the results of his experiment from the outset: The two hair-bearing plugs from the hairy part of the scalp grew hair whether they were transplanted into the hair-bearing or the bald part of the scalp, while the two plugs taken from the bald part of the scalp did not grow hair no matter where they were planted.

Orentreich had shown undeniably that a plug of hair cut from hair-bearing scalp would regrow and prosper in a part of the head long thought to be incapable of sprouting hair. And hair follicles that could not sprout hair could not be revived just by moving them to another part of the head.

He claimed in his paper that he was merely trying "to study some factors in the pathogenesis of certain dermatological disorders" and not invent a million-dollar industry. But of the sixty-five people in Orentreich's original study, fifty-two had male pattern baldness and Orentreich transplanted the hair, conveniently, along their receded hairlines.

He then did what any self-respecting scientist would do: He wrote it up for the journals.

"The grafts . . . continued to show hair growth [even during the] continued recession of the hairline," Orentreich wrote. "Moreover, the hair growth of the grafts appeared unimpaired." Those were the sentences that changed the world.

But the world wasn't ready for such a radical attack on nature (even though, in essence, that is what scientists do for a living). The *Archives of Dermatology*—the field's premier journal at the time— rejected Orentreich's results as "not possible."

"I still have the letter," said Orentreich, who still lives in New York, practices dermatology and performs hair transplants (his son, David, and daughter, Catherine, work alongside him at the sprawling fifty-person practice on Manhattan's tony East Side). "The editor of the journal was a friend of mine and he told me that when they sent out the study to be peer-reviewed, none of the other doctors could believe my results. They just said it was not possible to do that."

It wasn't until seven years later that Orentreich finally got the paper published in the *Journal of the New York Academy of Sciences*.

Even though the experiment was old by medical standards, the study was anything but stale in the medical community. Even seven years later, Orentreich was still breaking news about the possibility of hair transplants. Two years after that, the *Archives of Dermatology* finally saw the light, publishing a paper by another doctor who said he had also had success using Orentreich's technique. The revolution had come and, amazingly, it was still Orentreich's to lead.

And this is where everything went awry.

As an academic exercise, Orentreich's work was astounding. He had, simply put, invented a way of growing hair on a bald man's scalp. Even in his dry scientific language—"It is clear that possibly there may be far-reaching significance of the techniques used here," he wrote in that 1959 paper, underestimating the impact of what he'd done—you can tell that something was up.

So could anyone who read the paper. Orentreich was immediately flooded with calls, all from doctors who wanted to come to his clinic and learn the procedure (some of whom were bald and wanted to *volunteer* for the procedure, which they would also learn from the master and perform back in their own practices).

Orentreich was generous with his time, throwing open his practice to anyone who wanted to watch and learn the procedure.

"I had seventy-five physicians saying, 'If you can do this, do it for me,' " Orentreich recalled. "For the first two years, I was doing doctors for no charge. There were a lot of bald physicians for whom I did a frontal peak so they could show their patients. But before I knew it, my entire practice was being taken over by transplants. My life was becoming overwhelmed."

But Orentreich's generosity accomplished two things: It secured his reputation as an especially giving teacher while it also ensured that his technique—large, plug-style grafts—would be the industry standard for years.

Hindsight is twenty-twenty and there's no shortage of crusading hair transplant surgeons, consumer advocates and, in some cases, state attorneys general who are examining with keen eyes Orentreich's legacy: the work of some doctors still using his original techniques.

From the early 1960s until the mid-1980s, tens of thousands of men underwent hair transplant surgery with large grafts, paying large sums for the privilege and, in many cases, leaving their doctors' offices satisfied.

For decades, Orentreich's punch grafts were the state of the art of hair transplantation. The process was simple: a 4-millimeter hole punch, which looked about as sophisticated as a drill bit, was utilized to extract large plugs from the donor area. Then, the same punch created graft sites in the bald areas of the scalp.

The result? Dense grafts that looked good for a while—until a man's natural hair receded, leaving only the pluggy, doll's-head look of the punches. Although punch grafts are rarely used anymore, when people think of hair transplants, "plugs" are still what they think of. (On a telling episode of *Seinfeld,* the ever-picky romantic neurotic Elaine Benes dismisses an ardent suitor by describing his hair with the one-word expletive: "plugola.")

ABC News anchor Hugh Downs got his famous hair transplant during the large-plug era [http://www.abcnews.go.com/onair/2020/downs_hugh_bio.html]. Despite the fact that the plugs were noticeable, Downs told his viewers on *20/20* in 1985 that he had the procedure "because I felt unsure of my looks due to losing hair" and was thankful that he did. "I feel it's helped my confidence and I've been extremely pleased."

More and more customers kept rolling in, and the sound of a readily ringing cash register, whether you're a surgeon or a salesman (some are both), is a very persuasive argument against change.

Some people outside the hair transplant community saw what was going on even then. "Hair transplants are ugly, bloody and don't always work," Sandomir wrote in 1990. "Even when they do, they leave you with a head that looks like a bad corn crop in Nebraska after a drought."

But it's not clear how much Orentreich deserves these attacks. Again, the aluminum siding analogy is appropriate: Millions of people had their homes refurbished with the cheesy siding and were happy with the results—until something new, something more modern came along and made everything before it look old.

"The 4-millimeter plug that had been ordained as the optimal vehicle for moving hair was actually of a size that had no counterpart in nature," Robert Bernstein wrote in a journal article a few years ago that was highly critical of Orentreich's technique, though not the doctor himself, a thin line of criticism that Bernstein is constantly walking. "The decision to use 4-mm plugs was based mainly upon technical rather than aesthetic considerations," and it went unchanged "possibly because of Dr. Orentreich's deservedly high esteem in the medical community."

Even as late as 1985, Orentreich was still defending his procedure and the hand punch—named after him—that was still the instrument of choice.

"Punch graft hair transplantation is an efficacious procedure that will continue to be used until a safe and effective medication is devised to regrow the miniaturized follicles of male pattern baldness," he wrote. The words were outdated almost as he wrote them; such "medication" does not yet exist, but punch grafts have become obsolete, defying Orentreich's prediction.

Others were equally aggressive in defending the procedure. Hair transplant surgeon James Pinsky, a doctor's doctor, learned the Orentreich techniques early and defended the procedure as one that was not essentially for vanity, but to correct misperceptions.

To Pinsky, being bald is the same as having bags under your eyes, a common facial feature. People with bags are often told, "You look tired," when, in fact, they're not tired at all. Getting those bags removed, Pinsky argues, is not a case of vanity, but merely a way to no longer be viewed for what you are not. In the case of baldness, that means being viewed as being older than you are.

But Pinsky does plead guilty to partial vanity, admitting that an alternative to transplants—hairpieces—fails because wigs or toupees don't get to the central problem of hair loss: self-image. The hairpiece is so clearly not a part of its wearer that the man never gets to think of himself as "changed." He still can't look in the mirror and see himself.

And University of Pennsylvania dermatology professor Kligman championed the procedure—but cautioned that "surgical therapy of the excessively neurotic should be avoided, since their visions of a new, beautiful self can not be fulfilled."

Many hair transplant specialists go red when reminded of such comments because of the implication that unsatisfied customers must, inherently, be "excessively neurotic."

"Thousands of people were harmed by Norman Orentreich's clones," said a well-respected transplant surgeon who refused to give his name. "It's sad, because the story of hair transplants in the twentieth century is not Orentreich's discovery of the four-millimeter punch, but the discovery of the single follicular unit."

Medicine is fickle in that way. It's odd to think that Norman Orentreich's legacy could be seen as tainted. A member of fifty international dermatological, surgical and gerontological associations, Orentreich has published hundreds of papers on topics from hair transplants to pustular acne to liver function to miniature poodles (OK, only their skin). Much of his recent work has been ground-breaking in the understanding of why we age and how we can slow down that biological clock.

He is the founder of the Orentreich Foundation for the Advancement of Science. The American Geriatrics Society, which coined the term "gerontology," was founded by a group of experts on aging around a desk in his office. He has won scores of honors and held dozens of important titles. He owns six U.S. patents.

"He is a brilliant doctor," said O'Tar Norwood, a renowned hair transplant surgeon whose Norwood baldness classification system is still in use today [http://www.hairadvocates.com/nhscale.html].

But even Orentreich's biggest fans—Norwood learned hair transplantation in Orentreich's clinic—have cast doubt on the doctor's legacy.

"What's so stupid is that we were doing large grafts until 1985," Norwood said. "You can't take anything away from Norman Orentreich, but after he invented the procedure, he turned away from it rather than refining it."

David Orentreich defended his father's work—and, de facto, his own—by saying that large plugs were abandoned "very quickly" once it became clear that other doctors were getting better results with one-millimeter grafts and, eventually, single follicular units.

But his admission only highlighted the obvious: The revolution that Orentreich began in 1959 was "won" by others after the leader became obsolete, a Sun Yat-sen eclipsed by a Chiang Kai-shek.

"There is a reluctance to change, but that can be a healthy reluctance," David Orentreich told me during a break in a transplant he was performing on, oddly enough, his office manager.

"But I think this practice was open-minded because the goal was to get a better result for the patient. It wasn't hard for us to switch [to smaller grafts]. We made the transition as it was happening. Our reluctance was minimal."

Perhaps the most telling evidence is that there are no 4-millimeter punches in the drawers in Orentreich's operating rooms. Instead of fifteen to twenty hair grafts, his grafts are all single follicular units of one to three hairs, most implanted into a 1-square-millimeter hole. The largest punch he even has on hand is 2 square millimeters.

As a former patient, Gary Hitzig subscribes to Kligman's famous criticism of the "excessively neurotic" bald men who sometimes come in for hair transplants. "Some patients, like people with anorexia who can't help seeing a fat person in the mirror no matter how much weight they lose, will never be satisfied by hair transplants," said Hitzig.

Some doctors argue that those people are not good candidates for the procedure and should be turned away. Hitzig apparently operates on them anyway. And in some cases, it's come back to haunt him.

On the West Coast, the bad side of hair transplantation is represented ably by Dr. Larry Lee Bosley, one of the business's major marketers. Bosley has had his license temporarily suspended in more than a dozen states, most recently in California. Bosley and the California Medical Board are well acquainted, with charges of unlicensed medical practices and false advertising going back to 1979.

According to the California Medical Board, one of the "after" photos in Bosley's marketing material—captioned "Hairline after micrograft procedures"—was not of a patient at all, but of an employee who, the court papers charged, "had never undergone any hair restoration procedures."

In the most recent accusation against Bosley, the board accused him of continued false advertising ("after" photos were "altered, airbrushed and/or otherwise retouched," the state charged) and unlicensed practices involving the use of "senior medical consultants" who were neither senior, nor medical.

Worse, the board alleges, one patient lay on the operating table for five hours before a doctor finally came in and closed the gaping wound from his donor site.

"Such conduct . . . constitutes unprofessional conduct and gross negligence," California charged.

As in prior cases, Bosley, who denies any wrongdoing, reached a settlement with the board that included payment in excess of $600,000 but allowed him to continue practicing.

In the past, when such heat was on, many doctors—especially cosmetic surgeons—circled the wagons. A few years ago, when a lawyer took out large ads in several New York papers to solicit dissatisfied hair transplant clients for a lawsuit, one hair transplant doctor went so far as to gather a dozen of his competitors at his house to devise a strategy to combat the coming malpractice suits.

"What are we going to do?" the doctor asked, according to someone who was there.

There was much grumbling about how lawyers had turned satisfied customers into unsatisfied plaintiffs. There was a lot of whining about how doctors were being persecuted by patients who expected too much and ambulance chasers who'd do anything for a buck.

But even though the meeting had been convened as a way of defending the status quo, things started to change.

"They realized if they kept doing what they were doing, there would continue to be lawsuits," said a doctor who was there. "So they actually started doing better work."

This new leaf got turned just as Texas-based surgeon Bobby Limmer, Robert Bernstein and others were leading the campaign to graft only single follicular units rather than larger punches.

Today, grafts are dissected under a microscope to avoid separating hairs from those follicular units, which consist of the hair shafts, a band of collagen called the perifolliculum, sebaceous glands, connective tissue, a vellus follicle and a neurovascular plexus in one compact hexagonal unit. Follicular units are spaced evenly across the scalp, about one unit for every square millimeter.

Follicular units weren't discovered until well into the hair transplant era. In 1984, a histologist named J. T. Headington transected a piece of scalp horizontally at the sebaceous gland level and put it under an electron microscope, only to discover that single hairs were not equally spaced all over the head, but clustered in these equally spaced single- and multihair units.

That put the entire hair transplant business—and it *is* a business—on a collision course with the future.

The 1984 study was groundbreaking in terms of providing surgeons with a new understanding of how the scalp works and how the hair grows naturally. It doesn't grow in large punches—that much everyone knew—but surgeons were reluctant to do anything else because smaller grafts meant more time, which in turn meant fewer patients could be seen and that more staff would be needed, which in turn meant less profit for the practice.

"No one in the hair transplant world paid any attention to Headington because he was a pathologist, not a dermatologist," Bernstein said.

Subsequent studies have shown that hairs separated from their follicular units don't grow back as well. And by maintaining the integrity of the follicular units, hair docs minimize the risk of having hairs growing in the wrong direction or separating families of hairs behind a surgical version of the Berlin Wall.

"That's how nature creates density," says Michael Reed, showing me what follicular units look like under the microscope, like villages in rural areas seen from an airplane. "If you had follicular units with only one hair, we'd all be born with see-through hair. At the periphery of the scalp, the units are single or double and they tend to be finer. In the denser areas, the hair shafts themselves are denser and coarser and are bundled in larger numbers."

Ever since abandoning plug grafts, Robert Bernstein has always worked with the outspoken passion of a recovering addict. As a dermatological resident in the late 1970s at Albert Einstein College of Medicine, he was taught the Orentreich technique, featuring slightly smaller, but still grotesque, 3-millimeter punches.

"I did a few of them as a resident, but the procedure was so bad that I stopped doing them," he said. But even as his own hair-transplant-free dermatology practice grew, Bernstein kept up with the latest literature, hoping to someday offer an improved procedure to patients who asked for it.

"I went back into the business [in 1994] because transplants had gotten better," Bernstein said. "You could do good work and have satisfied patients."

Reed, who was a dermatological resident at New York University around the same time as Bernstein was at Einstein, is in the same camp. By the time he got out of medical school, Reed was offered a full-time job in NYU's pharmacology faculty. But when the doctor who ran the hospital's renowned hair loss clinic retired, Reed was asked to run it.

"I didn't volunteer, I was drafted," Reed said. "I wouldn't have gone into hair loss on my own. But I ran the clinic for three years and we were doing the old plug-type transplantations. I didn't like the technique that much, but in the nineties, it started getting better. We had better equipment, better ways of making grafts, more journals devoted to the subject, and I evolved with my field."

Like Bernstein, Reed's orientation to his field is primarily academic, not commercial (although both make good livings planting good hair into bald scalps). And Reed also blasts doctors who didn't "evolve."

"In the past, when patients were unhappy with the results of their plug transplants, the solution was doing more work," he said. "The only thing that got better was the doctor's bank account. The patient got worse and worse."

But with techniques having improved, Reed is comfortable that his practice is about 60 percent hair transplants, 40 percent general and cosmetic dermatology (which, as any Manhattanite knows, probably typically means taking pimples off the faces of spoiled rich kids, performing liposuctions and injecting Botox, a form of botulism, to paralyze and smooth the age lines on the faces of the ladies who lunch).

It's a good practice and Reed has a well-deserved good reputation. Or, as his receptionist gushes, "He doesn't just suck fat! He sculpts the body!"

"To be honest," Reed admits, "it's more fun to do liposuction than hair transplants because it's instant gratification. The day after a liposuction, the patient looks great." Hair transplants rarely look good after one 500-graft session. And even when they do, more sessions are needed as the patient's natural hairline recedes, leaving only the transplanted hair.

Where Reed is satisfied with the state of the business, Bernstein is still the field's angry middle-aged man. Through his journal articles—he writes about a dozen a year, a remarkable output for someone who works twelve hours a day in his Fort Lee, New Jersey, clinic—Bernstein has established a deserved reputation for never being satisfied.

When Hitzig, for example, published a paper in a hair transplant journal rechristening his "slot graft" technique as "follicular unit coupling," Bernstein's response was swift and to the point. While never mentioning Hitzig by name, Bernstein condemned him for trying to jump on the "follicular unit bandwagon."

" 'Follicular unit coupling' is an interesting choice of terminology," Bernstein wrote sarcastically. "What will be next? According to this article, we should probably rename Orentreich's original punch-graft method 'cylindrically bundled follicular unit transplantation.' . . . Re-working the name of the slot graft technique takes us back to the '60s, when we used to put Mercedes hood ornaments on the front of a Volkswagen. . . . A slot by any other name is still a slot."

Bernstein still claims he does not want to be the policeman of the hair transplant industry, but admits his approach "has pissed off some people."

"I write articles criticizing specific techniques, not specific doctors," he says. "I've been accused of being a zealot, but I want the profession to do well. I believe that hair transplantation can work and can make people's lives better. But we would all be multimillionaires if we all did good work. The biggest threat to me comes not from my competition but from my competition doing bad work. That hurts all of us."

Several times a week, Bernstein repairs a competitor's botched work on one of Kligman's "excessively neurotic" people, victims of bad grafts whose heads resemble the comic-book stereotype of a bad transplant. To make the much-needed repair, Bernstein removes the graft whole, dissects it into four or so follicular units apiece, and then transplants the new grafts into other areas of the balding scalp.

"There are doctors out there who are still doing this to patients!" Bernstein thunders.

Fellow surgeon Dow Stough, whose father, Bluford Stough, learned the procedure from Orentreich himself, was a bit more diplomatic. "Now we know that the key is a natural look rather than just building a wall of large grafts."

At a recent symposium at New York's Plaza Hotel, Stough talked of plug grafts in the same way that historians talk about the days when amputations were done without anesthesia, acknowledging the error but implying that bad work could not be avoided due to lack of established alternatives. Plug transplants are not ancient history, however, but modern case studies. Patients that Bernstein refers to as "maimed" or "butchered," Stough euphemistically calls "those poor, unfortunate souls who received the benefit of what we did twenty years ago."

One of those souls belongs to John Ricotta, a salesman from Knoxville, Tennessee, whose head is a veritable archaeological site tracing the very history of hair transplantation from the late 1960s to today.

Ricotta has no regrets about all the work he's had done—some of it good, some of it very, very bad—but he knows his head could be the centerpiece of an entire semester at medical school.

There are the large-plug grafts from his first transplant, back in the 1960s. There's the longitudinal scar from his scalp reduction, a popular "face-lift for the scalp" that was widely performed in that era. There are the plugs from his second transplant. There are the shotgun harvesting scars on the back of his head. And there are the single follicular units that Bernstein has put in to re-create a natural hairline.

It's amazing, but at long last, he actually looks good.

"I have no regrets," said Ricotta, who underwent the repeated procedures because he felt he needed to look younger. "I always had whatever technique was available at the time. Sometimes it came out looking good, sometimes not."

Ricotta admits he "looked a little pluggy," but it was never a problem until his natural frontal forelock finally receded. That's when he came to Bernstein for a new hairline.

How a Knoxville salesman ended up in the office of a New Jersey dermatologist who doesn't widely advertise offers a telling glimpse into a business that is still without a code of standards or a uniform set of ethics.

"I went to a transplant guy in Nashville to see if he could fill in my hairline," Ricotta said. "He looked at the back of my scalp and said, 'I don't think I can take any more plugs from your donor site.' He actually said 'plugs.' Can you believe that some doctors are still doing plugs? I heard him say that and I knew I needed to find someone else."

Consumer advocate Spencer Kobren, whose book *The Bald Truth* is a bible for anyone considering covering, medicating or surgically altering his bald head, complained that hair transplantation won't get much better until it's no longer treated as a business.

"It is not so much a *medical specialty,* one that serves *patients,* but a *business* that serves *consumers,*" he said.

And that's why the dedicated hair transplant surgeons and their technicians cut the donor site into follicular units, the naturally occurring groups of one, two, three or four hairs that become clear only under the microscope.

—

While Reed's technicians cut their grafts, Tony is having a snack and watching a videotape of *The Big Chill,* a film that centers around a group of aging baby boomers as they confront the mediocrity and shattered dreams of their middle age—an ironic pick for a guy undergoing a procedure to cure a particularly common ravage of middle age.

The first cuts divide the donor strip of 1,500 hairs into small blocks of fatty tissue that each look like a hairy pat of butter or a theatrical mustache Vincent Price would've worn. (Some technicians liken it to caterpillars or sushi.)

From those strips, technicians will keep cutting until they have hundreds of follicular unit grafts—each of which contains one to four hairs—ready for insertion.

Larry Leonard is one of Reed's technicians. A veteran of other practices, he's seen the worst hair transplantation has to offer: the factorylike speed of some of the industry's physician-businessmen, the shoddy surgery, the grafts wasted due to mishandling.

Dissection of the donor site is the most painstaking part of the entire procedure. For an hour and a half—as Tony watches everything from the funeral that brings together all the old college friends to *The Big Chill*'s sex-filled climax—Leonard and Olinsky use a stereomicroscope to help them cut away extra scalp tissue with a simple razor blade and arrange their grafts in petri dishes containing one-, two-, three- and four-haired units, as well as a few grafts of two follicular units.

It is exacting but not difficult work, and as I watch, I am reminded of assembly-line workers, in whose hands is left the job of building the machine even though they had no role in its design. In many ways, theirs is the most important part of the process, yet it involves the brain the least, the closest thing to monkey work that surgery has to offer.

The technicians have different ways of achieving the same result: Leonard lines up his grafts on a moistened tongue depressor so they resemble Russian missiles in a 1961 spy satellite photo of Cuba, while Olinsky prefers to push all her grafts into a pile and then spill them in a saline-filled petri dish.

Meanwhile, Reed has the blue Sharpie out again, this time to trace a line along Tony's scalp, where he will soon have a hairline again. Like most doctors, Reed resists his patients' persistent call to have the hairline lower than it should be. Bald men, it seems, are so excited about the return of hair to the front of the head that they forget that they will look ridiculous if their hairline extends down to the bridge of their nose.

Reed makes two or three test punches into Tony's scalp. Satisfied, he starts making punches in a pattern that resembles the dotted line on a coupon, each hole trickling a tiny amount of blood. The triangular punch, whose incision resembles the Mercedes-Benz logo, makes a disquieting sound as it enters the skin, much like the fleshy thud you hear when you poke the sharp end of a knife into a raw breast of chicken.

After finishing a front row, he makes three more before moving to a slightly larger punch to create holes he'll later fill with two-follicular-unit grafts, following the hair transplant world's conventional wisdom: small, single hair grafts up front, to create a natural-looking hairline; larger, double- and triple-hair grafts behind to create density.

A nurse uses a metal clicker to count off all the holes he has made into Tony's head, an unnerving clicking that contrasts with the dull punching sound Reed makes with the triangular tool.

Almost unnoticed, oddly, is the patient, who is meant to just sit there and take it. With all the anesthesia, all he hears is the sound of the punch going into his scalp, but he doesn't know what he's hearing because the scalp is such an imperfect conductor of sound.

"Is that popping sound the scalpel hitting my skull?" Tony asks.

"No, no, we're not going *that* deep," Reed assures him.

When the counter gets to 430 or so, Reed is satisfied that he's created the makings of a first-class head of hair.

Now he has to work fast.

Because hair grafts are living tissue, the goal is to get them into the patient's head as quickly as possible, lest they dry out and be unable to survive the regrowth process. Reed dampens a circular piece of gauze, tapes it onto the back of his hand and loads it up with grafts.

With fifty or so on his hand, Reed barely has to move to get his next graft, a key timesaver. Leonard prefers to have ten grafts stuck onto his index finger.

Although Reed is diligent and careful, there is something less than dainty about the surgery I am witnessing. Reed grabs each graft from the bottom with jeweler's forceps and basically shoves it into the hole, bulb first, working it down with tweezers in the other hand. I like this technique better than pushing the graft into the hole, but it still looks haphazard and sloppy.

*The Big Chill* has started over again and Leonard, still in his twenties, can't place the movie's opening song, "You Can't Always Get What You Want."

"It's the Rolling Stones!" Reed says, picking another two-hair graft from the moistened pad. "I can't believe you don't know the Rolling Stones."

"Well," Leonard answers, loading up more grafts on his index finger. "At least I know transplanting."

Through all the commotion of two men sticking tissue into his head, Tony falls asleep and begins snoring. He's missing quite a show. With so many grafts so close to each other—and with the scalp as flexible as a big sheet of rubber—it's sometimes tough to get them to stay in place. Like roasted garlic cloves being squeezed out of their skin or a bookshelf with too many paperbacks on it, grafts will sometimes pop out if another graft is inserted too close. A great deal of Reed and Leonard's time is spent cajoling grafts back into place.

After an hour and a half of pushing and pulling hairs, the work is done. Tony is wrapped up in antibiotic-treated gauze, which is tied under his chin so the bandage doesn't slip when he sleeps. He ends up looking like a guy in a Marx Brothers comedy who's just had brain surgery.

When Tony leaves, Reed has a chance to reflect on the job. He feels in some way that his entire profession is changing, that he is treating the last generation of men who do not have to go bald because of their genetic predisposition.

"Propecia does arrest hair loss," Reed says. Of course, he knows that the drug doesn't work for every man—and even the ones for whom it would work are most likely not even interested in treating their baldness.

But for Tony, who doesn't want to take medication for the rest of his life, Reed bought him a few years he would not have had. When Tony's natural hairline recedes, he'll still have the frontal forelock that Reed just transplanted, the Paul who's been paid after the mugging of Peter.

The forelock is the key, Reed believes, because as long as you still have some hair in the middle of your temporal region, people looking at your head will not perceive you as bald—even if everything beyond that is a desert of defoliated scalp.

"That forelock will stand alone," Reed says, tired from a day's work. "And it will look OK because it exists in nature."

*Chapter 7*

—

# A TALE OF TWO DRUGS:
# ROGAINE AND PROPECIA

"In truth, a mature man who uses hair-oil, unless medicinally, that man has probably got a quoggy spot in him somewhere. As a general rule, he can't amount to much in his totality."
—HERMAN MELVILLE (1819–91), author of *Moby-Dick*

They didn't know what they had.

The scientists at the Upjohn Company in Kalamazoo, Michigan, weren't trying to cure baldness in 1960. They were looking for something a little more beneficial to society, a way of reducing hypertension. In fact, they weren't looking at baldness at all (except when they looked in the mirror, perhaps)—but baldness came looking for them.

Upjohn's happenstance development of the most important treatment for hair loss since the invention of the wig in 3000 B.C. is not merely a story of a group of clever scientists, but also a glimpse into a rarely seen—and underappreciated—facet of medical research: chance.

In a modern world such as ours, coincidence is not something that we expect in our scientific research. Sure, we cherish the apocryphal tale of how a New England housewife accidentally spilled bits of chocolate into her cookie batter to create the Toll House cookie and we venerate what happened when a bunch of stoned-out hippies sold about two thousand tickets to a little arts and folk music fest called Woodstock—but from our scientists, we expect precision.

We expect hypotheses that get proven—or don't—and lead to established facts that become part of our academic canon. We like things cold and clean and logical.

We don't expect a blood pressure medication to start growing hair unless we theorize beforehand that it *will* grow hair.

"But you have to realize, this is how many drug uses were discovered," said Taft "Mac" Corum, who recently retired after thirty-one years at Upjohn (now officially known as Pharmacia & Upjohn). "Whenever scientists worked with a new compound, they'd put it through various pharmacologic screens to see what it would do. If it showed some action, they'd do some more tests. But that doesn't mean they knew why it did whatever it did. Remember, they didn't know how aspirin worked for the first ninety years it was around."

By comparison, the scientists at Merck knew from the outset that their prostate medication, Proscar, could grow hair—but they didn't care.

Before clinical trials reported that patients were growing hair, researchers at the New Jersey–based pharmaceutical giant knew that the same biological processes that enlarge the prostate—namely, the metabolism of testosterone into DHT by the enzyme 5-alpha reductase—also shrink hair follicles.

But they were too busy worrying about enlarged prostates—a condition called benign prostatic hyperplasia (BPH), which affects almost all men—to care about the scalp.

"From a medical standpoint, it would have been irresponsible to develop a drug for male pattern baldness before the drug to treat BPH," said Merck's Keith Kaufman, a senior director for clinical research. "But we had known since 1974 that male pattern baldness and benign prostatic hyperplasia were caused by the same thing."

It's a tale of two drugs.

If the best way to a man's heart is through his stomach, it may also provide the ideal route to his scalp. Upjohn's gastroenterological research unit was merely looking for a drug that could fight ulcers when it happened upon a compound called N,N-diallylmelamine (DAM). Researchers found that it didn't do much for stomach ailments, but it did prove to be great at relaxing the walls of blood vessels.

The compound was then punted to the company's cardiovascular research unit, which checked out the drug for hypertension. When early experiments failed to show any reduction in hypertension, scientists synthesized new versions of the molecule. This time, it seemed to work in animal studies, but when the compound was tested in humans in 1961, two people ended up giving their lives to medical science. To add insult to surgery, a few dogs presented with heart lesions as a result of taking the compound.

"Now the reputation of this potential drug had already been damaged," the late Gerald Zins, who worked on the drug at the time, wrote a few years back.

Upjohn's efforts were, to say the least, set back and the company withdrew the hypertension drug—with its still-unknown hair-growing effect—in 1962. But the company did not give up.

Over the next six years, Upjohn synthesized hundreds of new analogs of DAM. The one that showed the most promise (i.e., fewer dogs complained of heart lesions) was called minoxidil.

Convinced it was onto something, Upjohn filed an Investigational New Drug Application in 1968.

The drug sailed through Phase I testing, which involves just a few doses of the medication to prove that the drug will not harm humans. It was only during Phase II clinical testing—when subjects are on the drug for months—that Upjohn started hearing reports of hair growth, with hair showing up on patients' backs, cheeks and sometimes even their heads.

But the studies were still in the hands of the cardiovascular researchers, who reacted to the sudden hair growth as would any researcher who had been looking for something else.

"To them, the side effect was totally unwelcome," Corum said. "They viewed it as something they needed to fix. You have to understand, they were cardiovascular researchers trying to get a drug through the approval process," not baldness researchers.

If it hadn't been for an Upjohn researcher named Carl Schlagel, minoxidil's hair-growing properties might have been "solved" and never heard from again. Luckily for bald men everywhere, Schlagel—who, it must be pointed out, suffered from thinning hair—saw lemonade in the cardiovascular researchers' lemon.

"Carl Schlagel was the champion of this drug," Corum said. "From the time he heard about minoxidil's hair growth, he became excited. No one in senior research management was keen on pursuing it, but Carl kept it alive."

From a coolly logical management perspective, there was no reason to bother with the hair-growing possibilities. This was the 1970s, long before the era of "lifestyle drugs" such as Viagra or Retin A. In those years, there was no such thing as a prescription cosmetic.

And if it hadn't been for Schlagel, there might never have been.

So unlike Merck's scientists, who put aside their compound's hair-growing potential so as not to interfere with the approval process of their prostate drug, Upjohn began pursuing the hair-growing side of their medication even while pursuing FDA approval for their blood pressure medication. Studies of topical applications of minoxidil began in 1971 and again showed promise.

"The ingredients for success were now assembled," Zins said. "We had a drug that caused hair to grow. . . . The more immediate obstacle we were facing, however, was to prove minoxidil's safety in sufficiently convincing terms."

That would have to wait until late 1977 because the hypertension-lowering oral minoxidil was still proving problematic in human testing (as a blood pressure medication, minoxidil was certainly a great baldness drug). Loniten, Upjohn's name for the blood pressure medication, was finally approved in 1979.

But it would take nine more years before the FDA would approve Rogaine (the name was chosen because the FDA rejected Upjohn's first choice, Regain, as misleading).

The FDA announcement of Rogaine's approval was issued in an August 18, 1988, press release written, as is typical among scientists, with tremendous understatement and restraint: "Because FDA has never previously approved such a product (despite a plethora of products claiming to be baldness cures), there is considerable interest in this one."

The FDA concluded that although "the product will not work for everyone," 39 percent of the men studied had "moderate to dense hair growth on the crown of the head."

Alex Busansky, now a lawyer with the Department of Justice, was still in law school when he signed up for one of Rogaine's early trials in 1986. For him, a man who flashed his hair like other men flash biceps, the drug was a godsend.

"I had great hair," Busansky said. "I had hair of the century. It was thick, it was plentiful and I would style it to great effect. So when I started to lose it, it really affected me, even though I clearly wasn't bald. I guess it's like when you have a pimple; you see it much bigger than anyone else sees it."

Busansky was in the clinical trial for about a year and saw great results, but stopped taking the drug as he began to come to terms with his own baldness. Once he was out of law school and working at a prestigious law firm, looking young actually was a detriment to working his way up the firm ladder.

"When you're in your twenties in law school and you go out at night, you don't see a lot of bald men around," Busansky said. "When you're in your thirties and you're working in a law firm in New York, you do. Suddenly, if you're bald, you start to fit in."

Besides, research shows that the "Rogaine regain" generally peaks at one year. After that, you'll keep the hair you have (as the Upjohn slogan goes), but that's about it.

Just as scientists don't fully understand exactly how the cells in the base of a hair follicle signal to other cells to initiate the growth, or anagen, phase of the hair cycle, the scientists who created Rogaine don't fully understand how it works.

This is also something we don't expect from our scientists—and they'll take great pains to make sure the word doesn't get out. In fact, it seemed to me that Ron Trancik, senior director of clinical and medical affairs for Pharmacia & Upjohn, would rather do anything than talk about whether his best researchers know how minoxidil works.

"Do we totally understand how *anything* works?" he asks, avoiding my question as we sit in the cafeteria at the company's world headquarters in Peapack, New Jersey. Trancik had suggested the cafeteria, away from the dermatology and hair textbooks that line the walls of his office and mock his efforts to fully explain the pharmacology of his star product.

"I won't say we don't understand how minoxidil works," he reiterates. "What I'm going to tell you is that we don't know *exactly* at the molecular or biochemical level what it does to influence the hair cycling process."

This is where science gets imprecise and sloppy, like the housewife accidentally spilling chocolate chips into her cookie batter. After the fact, she can say it was all by design, but she knows it wasn't and she may not even understand how the fortuitous accident happened.

Minoxidil is not Propecia, which was spun off from a prostate drug with a specific goal in mind—to arrest male pattern baldness. Merck's scientists knew what caused it—the conversion of testosterone to DHT—and they knew how to block the enzyme that did it.

But when minoxidil was initially being tested, the very enzymatic processes that control most of our biological functions were not fully understood, so that understanding how Rogaine works—really works—is something that can be determined only now, after the chocolate chips have already been baked in and the cookies offered to passing motorists with their change.

"Just as Propecia has a mechanism—blocking the conversion of testosterone to DHT—we believe minoxidil has a mechanism, too," Trancik says.

This much we know: The drug opens up blood flow to the hair follicles—which is never a bad thing, and, in fact, was one of the hair-growing strategies of the snake-oil salesman of the early part of this century (some of whom used hot peppers to irritate the scalp and cause blood flow). But beyond that, it's anyone's guess. Some of Upjohn's research indicates that minoxidil affects potassium channels in the hair follicles and the chemical signals sent from the dermal papilla cells to the dormant hair bulb that trigger the onset of the growth phase.

"Listen, even though we know that Propecia is a 5-alpha reductase inhibitor, we don't really know the signals and the processes by which it inhibits that enzyme," Trancik says, clearly frustrated. "The mechanism of minoxidil remains somewhat elusive, but it bugs me when people say 'You don't know how it works.' We do know that minoxidil is first metabolized into a sulfated form—minoxidil sulfate—before it can be used by the cell."

Across the hall, in the suite of offices reserved for the marketing people, there's an entirely different form of confusion. Just as the scientists don't know how Rogaine works, the marketing people don't know how to make it work for the company.

Rogaine is one of only two FDA-approved medications to cure baldness—a condition experienced by more than half the world's population—yet Pharmacia & Upjohn makes so little money on the product that at some point many people within the company wonder why the drug giant even bothers.

When I stopped by the office of marketing manager Tim Canning, the first place my eyes traveled was not on his slowly disappearing, Rogaine-treated bald spot, but on a wood totem on his desk that reads, "$200m × 2004." It's a reminder of the company's seriously optimistic hopes for the drug: $200 million in sales—which would represent almost a doubling of the market—by the year 2004.

"Two hundred million by 2004. That's our mantra," Canning says. "We call it a 'BHAG,' a big, hairy, audacious goal."

Growing the sales of such an established product—especially one that is available in its generic form even in its "extra strength" dosage—would be almost unprecedented. But it's Canning's job.

"It's been a difficult business," Canning says diplomatically. "If you look at the mighty Merck, there was a period there where they were spending one dollar in advertising for every dollar in sales.

They envisioned a four-hundred-million-dollar market for Propecia, but they just didn't get it."

Propecia's sales are roughly $100 million a year—impressive, but not nearly what Merck thought they'd be. In fact, the company recently discontinued direct-to-consumer ads, a principal marketing strategy that involves getting very vague information into the hands of consumers and telling them, "Ask your doctor." The ads—which showed a man constantly confronted by subtle images of his coming baldness, such as uncovered planetarium domes and wind-denuded dandelions—were killed because they were not working (some say they failed because many bald men thought they were ads for Rogaine).

But, like Trancik, Canning has drifted from discussing Rogaine. When I bring him back to the topic, he can only grumble about lost opportunities. Rogaine was first introduced as a prescription drug in 1988, but when it went over the counter in 1996, the FDA made the rare decision not to grant Upjohn a three-year exclusive against competition from generic drugmakers, claiming that the company did not need to do a significant amount of new clinical tests before shifting to nonprescription uses.

Upjohn protested but lost, and Rogaine was unable to hold off the generics. And then, when the company introduced its extra-strength, 5-percent-minoxidil version of Rogaine in late 1997—and started spending heavily to promote it—Propecia rained on the Upjohn parade. As of this writing in November 2000, extra-strength Rogaine is about to become available in its generic form, too.

Nearly a decade later, everyone at Upjohn points to the nonexclusive decision as the beginning of the end.

"This product demands a lot of contact with the consumer and a lot of direct marketing, which the generics don't do," Canning says. "People buy the generics and then don't follow up. If they were our customers, we'd be spending money to keep them in compliance. We tell them, it's a great product and it works if you use it twice a day, every day. If we had maintained our exclusive, we could've been making that pitch to every minoxidil user from the start and grown the market so that when the generics came in, they could have their twenty to thirty percent and we'd still have our fair share."

Rogaine's sales dropped 32 percent after 1996 when Propecia hit the market. Although Rogaine sales are holding steady against the pill, Canning can only wonder what might have been.

"It's been profit challenged," he admits (yes, he really said "profit challenged"). "For this brand to make money now, we have to be very prudent. At the end of the day, we have to show that marketing Rogaine is better for the company than just buying T-bills."

That's a hard thing to do when Rogaine is not the silver bullet men have sought for millennia. The clinical trials of Rogaine proved that it won't be effective for everyone—and even those for whom it works will grow only peach fuzz rather than a full head of hair.

What's worse, Upjohn's internal marketing studies show that Rogaine has a disastrously high dropout rate. In its earliest days, men seemed to rush into Rogaine—some feeling, as Canning says, "that it would grow a Chia Pet on their heads"—only to be disappointed. Now, many men abandon the somewhat unpleasant, twice-daily minoxidil massages if they don't see results right away because they sense, perhaps unfairly, that they will *never* see results.

Only 40 percent of men who buy an initial supply of Rogaine buy a second. In the end, only 22 percent of the original pool are still Rogaine customers after their fourth purchase, according to statistics compiled for Upjohn by Nielsen, the TV ratings people.

Another Upjohn survey tracked users' expectations against their experience with the product. The "satisfaction rate" numbers (i.e., the difference between high expectations and low performance) in the survey "aren't even close," Canning admits.

Even as he looks across his glass cubicle to his two coworkers and sees their bald spots shrink on a weekly basis, thanks to Rogaine, Canning gets marketing reports showing that 60 percent of customers are worried about side effects (even though the FDA says the worst that could happen is an irritated scalp). Others complain of the difficulty in sticking with the "twice a day, every day" program.

But fully 70 percent complain about the price—men, by and

large, say they are willing to spend $15 to $20 a month if a product works, which has forced the company to roll out lower prices.

"Until you have a product that can grow that Chia Pet on a bald head—it's not out there, by the way, and it's not in clinical trials, either—you need to keep costs at a level that the consumer says is fair," Canning says. Upjohn now charges $49.95 for the three-month supply—smack in the middle of that $15 to $20 range—and will knock $5 off its one-month starter kit.

The price cut makes it even harder for Canning to reach his "$200m × 2004" goal—the price cuts just took 5 percent from future sales.

And to go after a bigger market, both Merck and Upjohn are taking the Joe Camel approach: Get 'em while they're young, with ads that target men who have only just begun to go bald—like Merck's cheeky commercials with the omnipresent chrome domes.

"We know we have a leaky bucket," Canning says. "People drop out, so we have to keep filling the bucket with new customers and then we have to encourage them to balance their expectations so they remain customers."

It's an uphill battle in a country where careers, personal health and even marriage are seen as temporary commitments. Rogaine and Propecia both depend on purchasers who will treat their medication like their health club—devoting themselves to regular use and the understanding that results won't come all at once, but in a very slow, almost imperceptible procession. But if you stick with it, you'll see something in a year.

Of course, if Canning figures out how to convince people to stick with it, there are thousands of health clubs around the country who'd like to know the secret.

If the mood at Pharmacia & Upjohn seems gloomy, it isn't any merrier at Merck, which is also finding the market for its revolutionary baldness medication as stunted as the follicles it restores.

To date, the drug has been prescribed to more than 680,000 men—a tiny fraction of the estimated billion men worldwide who could benefit from the drug's hair-saving effect.

Like Upjohn, Merck has its own internal studies to explain why bald men aren't popping as many pills or rubbing in as much medicine as the companies had hoped. Of the fifty-two million American men over the age of eighteen who experience hair loss, Merck surveys show that only 10 percent want to do anything about it.

And, if health club memberships are any indication, only a fraction of that number will actually make a move to do anything about it.

And only a fraction of that fraction will actually stick with it. Everyone starts a diet on a Monday morning and abandons it by Tuesday afternoon.

It should come as no surprise that of the nearly $1.3 billion spent on "curing" baldness, a full $1 billion is spent on hair transplants— a procedure that, extending the metaphor, is to baldness medications what liposuction is to regular exercise and sensible diet.

It is the quick fix that Americans generally prefer to hard work, emotional commitment or reasonable expectations.

Results with Propecia are similar to those with Rogaine (although no clinician has ever tested the drugs, literally, head-to-head). For Rogaine, scientists found that nearly 80 percent of subjects observed new hair growth or stabilization and diminished hair loss. Twenty percent got no benefit.

In the original clinical trial of Propecia, testing 1,879 men ages eighteen to forty-one, 86 percent said they experienced either an increase in hair count or maintenance of the hair they had. Scientists trained in the study of hair put the figure closer to 48 percent—but 93 percent of the men who were taking the inert placebo experienced hair loss during the same period.

The drug works. But then again, Merck always knew it would, once they got around to developing it.

The Merck campus in Rahway, New Jersey, is more like a college campus in a small town than a drug research and manufacturing plant. As I was waiting for Keith Kaufman at the security gate (which itself resembles a small-town police desk), two men, their T-shirts drenched in sweat, returned to campus from a lunchtime

Frisbee game, two women pushed strollers, and two slacker types strolled, coffee cups in hand, as if relaxing between class.

The security guard called me "young fella."

There was not a tie to be seen anywhere (especially on Kaufman, the company's senior director for clinical research in endocrinology and metabolism).

After the lack of a tie, the next thing you notice about Keith Kaufman is his hair. It is unavoidable. Kaufman has lots and lots of hair, a manly mixture of steel gray and pig-iron black. This is not hair that comes from hair transplants or drug protocols. This is hair that cascades, that waves across the forehead like the wing of a B-52. Kaufman's is a veritable seder plate of hair that he wears long in the front and so long in the back that he resembles guitarists from the Eagles in the post-hippie, "hair peace" days of the mid-1970s [http://www.eaglesmusic.com/gallery/bwcover.html].

Not only do bald men want this man's drug, they want his hair.

Kaufman joined Merck on Monday, October 7, 1991—a date emblazoned in the brain under all that hair because it was the same day that the company convened a meeting to design the first Phase II study of finasteride, the active ingredient in what would one day become Propecia.

Kaufman was in charge of getting Propecia tested and ready to be approved by the FDA—a follow-up to Proscar, the prostate version, which would get its federal stamp of approval in 1992.

Unlike Upjohn, Merck knew it would discover a hair-growing side effect to Proscar when it began its clinical trials. It all stemmed from two landmark papers in 1974 that reported on a rare group of men in the Dominican Republic who lacked the 5-alpha reductase enzyme that converts their testosterone into DHT. As a result, the men neither developed benign prostatic hyperplasia nor went bald. Just as Hamilton's castrata studies proved the link between male sex hormones and baldness, these studies showed the true culprit was testosterone's metabolized form, DHT.

Merck scientists were already working on androgen metabolism, Kaufman said, so when the journal articles appeared, they had the jump on other drug companies in trying to find an external method of mimicking the Dominican men's genetic inability to make DHT. Prevent DHT formation, and benign prostatic hyperplasia—and, don't forget, male pattern baldness—would be a thing of the past.

"There was no therapy for an enlarged prostate at that time except surgery," Kaufman said. "So our priority was clearly to study the prostate and get a drug approved before moving on to the baldness side. Once we understood the safety profile of finasteride and were comfortable with it, then we could take a look at the drug for another indication. Male pattern baldness was a worthy indication, but only after the prostate."

That type of risk assessment is common in the drug-approval process. In fact, other companies saw hair-growing side effects in their own drugs but intentionally passed up the chance to be the first drug company on the block with a Rogaine or a Propecia.

Hoffman-LaRoche, one of the biggest drug companies in the world, knew that its own hypertension drug was showing hair growth in clinical trials, but consciously avoided exploiting that side of the research.

"With drugs, you're always thinking about the risk/reward equation," said Herb Conrad, who was president of Roche's pharmaceutical division when the hair-growing hypertension drug was in the pipeline.

"When developing drugs, you're willing to take greater risks if the condition that is being cured is serious, such as heart disease or cancer. But baldness does not qualify in that way. No drug in development is perfectly safe, so you won't take that risk for a baldness treatment."

And there's a cost-benefit analysis for the company, as well. Where Upjohn saw a vast market to be tapped, Roche saw headaches. Conrad seemed to relish the fact that Rogaine "has not exactly been a blockbuster" for Upjohn—and remembered thinking at the time that even though he's bald, he wouldn't take a drug to prevent further hair loss. He doesn't think that influenced the company's decision not to pursue a hair-growth drug, but he can't be sure.

"In the end, we just didn't think strongly about it," Conrad said. That same risk/reward equation motivates his thinking today in his new role as chairman of GenVec, a company that is bringing to market several cutting-edge gene-therapy treatments.

The company's medical director, Ronald Crystal, has shown that he can use gene therapy to grow hair in mice—but Conrad and his board are not about to take the risk of exploiting gene-therapy techniques, which are still quite risky, simply to remedy a mildly annoying—though medically benign—cosmetic defect.

Instead, GenVec's first product will be a gene-therapy approach to growing new blood vessels in the heart, and its second will involve a new cancer treatment. If a mistake is made and someone dies as a result of a search for a cure for cancer, that can be justified. If someone dies during a trial for a baldness cure, "we would be vilified and rightly so," Conrad said.

But once Proscar was proven safe, Keith Kaufman of Merck says, "it would have been inappropriate *not* to look into the commercial opportunities of a baldness treatment."

Talking to Kaufman—and the dozens of other highly trained researchers, doctors and academics involved in ridding mankind of baldness—it is surprising to so rarely hear any laments at lives devoted to hair loss. One expects to find the best doctors seeking the most important cures. Just as TV medical dramas like *ER* never seem to focus any attention on, say, the hospital's dermatology clinic, one expects that doctors who work in the trenches of baldness have trouble feeling satisfied at the end of a day of performing a tiny piece of an experiment seeking to accelerate hair growth in a mouse.

"For me, no matter what research you're doing, you're trying to answer a scientific question," Kaufman says. "We've done a lot, but we still have yet to answer the question, 'Why does person A go bald and person B does not?' We know that it has to do with genetics, but we don't know where the genetic switches are. We don't know which proteins are the ones that cause the follicles to shrink. When we do, we can target drugs to stop that process."

So he's not really studying baldness; he's studying the basic genetic code of human life as it applies to one particular organ: the hair. Cracking that code, as many researchers are trying to do, will yield a wealth of information about other diseases and conditions.

A rationalization? Not entirely. Even though he's worked on drugs to prevent premature labor in women, forestall urinary incontinence or prevent prostate cancer, Kaufman always comes back to his work on Propecia.

"Look, this is not curing cancer, but this is very important to the men we're treating. I don't think I would've liked to lose my hair at age twenty-five." (One thing is sure: He'd look very, very different.)

Trancik, at Upjohn, agrees. Beyond the fact that the hair follicle is "a phenomenal organ to study," he believes that the psychological component to male or female pattern baldness make it every bit an important illness.

"Yeah, people don't take hair seriously, especially the counterparts to the FDA that have to approve our drugs overseas," he said. "They ask why we're wasting our time on this. But people have committed suicide because of their hair. And women with cancer have said no to chemotherapy because they don't want to lose their hair."

# Chapter 8

—

# THE "RALPH NADER OF HAIR"

"RESPECTABILITY, n. The offspring of a liaison between a bald
head and a bank account."
— AMBROSE BIERCE, *The Devil's Dictionary* (1911)

Mike, on the phone from New Jersey, just wants to know if
there's any hope for him.

It's after midnight on a Sunday night, a time when most men are
asleep with their lover beside them or resting up after a weekend
spent trying to satisfy certain needs that seem to gain in urgency as
the week speeds closer to Friday and Saturday nights.

But no, Mike hasn't been out on the town and he's not in bed with
a friend. The clock says it's late and when you're awake this late, the
mind plays tricks on you, convincing you that small problems are
big and big problems are surmountable only through the purchase of
a wide range of inscrutable products that, as luck may have it, are
sold at the very hours when a man's defenses are down and his self-
image rattled.

But Mike, who is forty-five and going bald, is trying to combat
the instinct to give in to the shameless come-ons and the commercial siren songs of the modern-day shysters. At this hour, other than
paying $3 a minute on a sleazy 1-900 line, Mike knows there's only
one place a man in his condition can go for comfort.

"Hi, Spencer, thanks for taking my call," he says, addressing
Spencer David Kobren, host of "The Bald Truth Radio Hour," a nationwide broadcast that Kobren says "separates the hope from the

hype in this unregulated industry." [http://www.thebaldtruth.org/html/radio_shows.htm]

"The Bald Truth" is also dedicated to the proposition that all bald men are created equal and that they are designed by their creator with one unalienable right: to be comforted and respected.

Kobren, whose own hair loss led him to drop everything he was doing professionally and begin an odyssey of research that resulted in his bestselling book, *The Bald Truth: The First Complete Guide to Preventing and Treating Hair Loss,* is just the man for the job. A New Agey, bead-wearing peacenik, Kobren mixes just the right amount of hard facts and soft emotion to give bald men a place where they can drop the macho mask they wear in the locker room or the chat room and lay down on a figurative couch with a box of Kleenex beside them.

So when Mike sheepishly—very sheepishly—tells Kobren that he's "lost quite a bit" of his hair, Kobren doesn't first dive into a long speech about a number of different products, some FDA approved, others not, that could work. No, Kobren wants to first understand who Mike is and what's on his mind.

The tone is pure therapy—not radio therapy, but real, honest concern.

"When did you start losing your hair, Mike?" Kobren asks. In most cases, he'll also ask, "How did that make you feel?" And he always calls everyone "friend" and urges them to "stay strong."

Mike says that he's not happy about his receding hairline—it makes him feel older and less attractive—but he doesn't know what to do. The Rogaine he's been using does not seem to work for him.

But he's obviously not given up entirely; after all, he's made this call, hasn't he? Kobren knows that—and it is that tiny ember of hope that he tries to stoke.

Rogaine is one of the few products that Kobren will allow to advertise on his show—which he controls entirely, because he pays for the airtime in about a dozen cities nationwide—but he is credible enough that he won't defend the somewhat-successful product when it cannot be defended.

"Rogaine does not work for everyone, but I want you to know, Mike, that there is hope," Kobren says, evoking that word again. Kobren proceeds to remind Mike that Propecia, the only other FDA-approved medication for baldness, is often successful, as are a number of nonmedicinal treatments, such as the extract from saw palmetto berries or a new product called Revivogen, the only non-FDA-approved product that he will allow to advertise on his show [http://www.revivogen.com].

But Mike has heard Kobren talk about such methods of preventing further hair loss. This time, it seems, he just needed the pep talk, the shoulder rub, the word "hope" echoing through the static.

"Good luck, buddy," Kobren says before taking his next call from Phil from Downey, California.

And so it goes for an entire hour, Kobren filling a void that exists for bald men in a world of product pushers, misinformation and doctors uninterested both in men's hair loss and the psychic cost it extracts. But Kobren is not playing a role. In a spiritual sort of way, he really does believe that hope works.

"The mind's ability to play a role in illness and recovery is entirely underestimated by modern science," he says. "I hear how doctors treat patients. If someone has a twenty-to-sixty-percent chance of survival, they say 'You have a twenty percent chance.' Well, sometimes you have to give people hope and they don't."

A few years ago, Spencer David Kobren was just another schlub losing his hair. He was twenty-two and, like many men with thinning hair, didn't like what he saw in the mirror every morning. Kobren also didn't like what he saw from the medical profession: lies, grandiose promises, useless products, lack of concern. Like many bald men, he tried everything—he remembers using inert products such as the Helsinki Formula and KeraKare, having hormone injections into his scalp and even checking out pulsed electrostatic-field barrages (a once-promising, now-ridiculed treatment)—but was always disappointed and always a few hundred bucks poorer. He used Rogaine, although he found that it didn't work for him as well as it had for all the men in Upjohn's "after" photos. The medication bought him some time, but didn't give him the thick head of hair he wanted.

Now, most men in that situation grumble to themselves at their naïveté and move on. It's been well documented in academic research that men are much more likely to sit idly by after being ripped off or disappointed than women, who are much more apt to complain and fight. Several hair transplant surgeons, for example, have told me of patients who, after suffering through a horrible transplant, merely start wearing hats rather than get the work repaired and their self-image restored. They were so disappointed in *themselves* for being taken that they couldn't even direct their ire toward the more appropriate target, the doctor.

But Kobren and his hairline refused to go quietly. With a background in the world of HMOs—he managed a program that provided homebound seniors with basic medical care such as blood pressure screenings and also managed two HMO facilities in New York—Kobren saw the medical profession at its money-hungry worst.

"Part of my job was to create reasons to perform basic diagnostic testing on seniors in order to bill Medicare," he said. "It was, in fact, good for the patients, but not good for the system. My outreach program billed Medicare more 'visits' in the first year than the first five years the HMO was in business."

What he learned was that "commerce is absolutely the number-one priority in health care today," he said. "The patient is of little concern. 'First, do no harm' has turned into 'Show me the money.' "

And the experience also taught him that medical fraud is easiest to perpetrate on the ignorant.

He set out to educate himself. Unable to find a medication that would retard his hair loss, Kobren first investigated hairpieces, surmising that he might someday be more than a curious bald man; he'd someday be a client. At the time, some companies were still sewing hairpieces onto the scalp with a kind of "belt loop" made of flesh. Other companies were sewing hairpieces directly into the scalp, a practice that is now illegal in most states. And most were just selling garbage, ill-fitting skullcaps that could be called "rugs" were it not unfair to the nation's legitimate carpeting industry.

"I saw it all, the hard sell, the deceptive marketing," he said. "The bottom line is that a hairpiece is a hairpiece, no matter how it's presented. There are good ones and bad ones, but they are all basically the same, a bunch of hair attached to a base that is attached to a balding scalp."

This was not an industry with the most sophisticated ethical code. Kobren did discover that some companies—such as the Hair Club for Men—made and marketed a legitimate product. He made a note of it; it might be useful in the future.

Subsequent personal investigation led him to his own experience with Propecia, the Merck drug that saves endangered hair follicles by reducing levels of dihydrotestosterone (DHT) in the bloodstream. Kobren "discovered" Propecia in 1994 when *The New York Times* ran an article about a Merck prostate drug that prevented testosterone from converting into DHT and had an interesting side effect: hair growth. A half dozen years of research had taught Kobren the link between hair loss and DHT, so he correctly surmised that a prostate drug that inhibited DHT production could have vast potential.

That drug, Proscar, had only just come on the market and clinical trials had just recently begun for Propecia, the lower-dosage, male baldness version of the drug. At that time, no doctor would prescribe Proscar for hair loss. Doctors are, generally speaking, reluctant to take the risk of prescribing even approved drugs for uses beyond their indications, unless, of course, a patient is suffering greatly.

Hair loss does not typically fall into that category—certainly not in pre-Viagra 1994, when "lifestyle" drugs were anathema to most physicians.

"There wasn't a doctor willing to let me take Proscar because I was too young to be experiencing any prostate problems," Kobren said. "They were concerned because if you take some prostate drugs for a long time, there's sometimes a feminizing effect. But I didn't want to wait until Propecia was fully tested. I wanted to take it *now.*"

Kobren found that other doctors—including the one who was

selling him a Rogaine–Retin A mixture—would always bad-mouth Proscar, as if they were more interested in preserving the status quo than actually making new, possibly superior treatments available to their patients.

But when he did his own research, Kobren discovered that the supposedly long list of side effects consisted only of five (which only a tiny percentage of men actually experienced, anyway). Oddly, the antidepressant that Kobren was taking (prescribed, he says, by a doctor who "thought that those not happy about losing their hair should cheer up about it") had sixty-one side effects—including hair loss!

Finally, Kobren convinced a doctor friend to write him a prescription.

"I said, 'Listen, I've been on antidepressants. If something goes wrong, I'll just stop taking the drug,' " Kobren recalled.

He didn't know it at the time, but Kobren was experiencing the exact mix of desperation, frustration, paranoia and anger that he so often hears from his radio show callers. He'd heard about a treatment, was denied it for reasons that seemed eminently logical to the person doing the denying, yet he still wanted it. Having experienced those emotions made Kobren empathetic in a way few else could be.

"I was not about to let someone control my destiny," he wrote in *The Bald Truth,* his tone almost exactly that of his callers. "I wanted to keep my hair, and I was willing to do anything that *I felt* was safe." (Emphasis added.)

He popped the first pill in December 1994 and guess what? Nothing went wrong. In fact, he saw a reversal in his hair loss within three months. Kobren was not remiss in thinking he was onto something. And if it worked for him, maybe it could work for others.

Few outside Merck knew that Proscar could be a significant hair loss medication, but Kobren saw the coming revolution in baldness. In 1996, before Propecia was approved, he started a rudimentary, text-only website—calling it "Major Hair Loss News"—that detailed his use of Proscar and, eventually, other information he'd discovered. Unlike doctors, Kobren could share all the information and let people make up their own minds.

"Ten thousand people came to that site, which, in 1996, was a lot," Kobren says today.

He pooled together all his research and sold it as an "information kit" for $5.95, to cover the postage and printing, he says.

"But I always said that if five ninety-five is a hardship, just send me a self-addressed stamped envelope," Kobren says. "I thought people would be too embarrassed not to send the money, but I was amazed at how many guys just sent the envelope. The newer bald guys sent the money, but the bitter guys didn't. I guess they'd been burned so many times by so many 'cures' that they didn't feel obligated."

One man—one of the guys who paid, apparently—even called him "the Hair Messiah."

And that's when Kobren knew he had found a new life's work: what he calls "consumer advocacy for the hair impaired."

Of course, continually reaching a wider audience has been a struggle all the way. After finding success with his website, Kobren shopped around a consumer bible–type book based on his investigations into all elements of the hair industry—medications, hair transplants, toupees and even nutrition.

He was turned down by thirty-three publishers. The publishing industry reacted to Kobren's proposal much as doctors react to men who complain about their baldness: *We'd rather spend our time on something more important.*

Someone in the book business apparently wasn't crunching the numbers. If even a small percentage of the 50 percent of men over age fifty who go bald would buy a book to learn more about their condition, some publisher would have a bestseller on his hands.

But no one was interested—until Merck got FDA approval to market Propecia. Suddenly, several publishers wanted to see "that bald book." The time was finally right.

Thanks to organizing his own book tours and speeches, Kobren has sold more than 650,000 copies of *The Bald Truth* since its initial publication in 1998. But when he tried to take the next step—a weekly radio show—he met the same resistance.

"They all wanted to know 'How are you going to keep the show going after the first month? What are you going to talk about?' " Kobren recalls. "I told them that two hundred thousand men are going to wake up tomorrow and see more hair in the drain. I'll be able to keep it going."

No radio stations would give him airtime, so he decided to buy it himself. In retrospect, that decision has served him well. By selling his own ads, Kobren gets a far greater degree of control than if he were merely an employee of a big radio station—and he gets to keep more of the profits.

Because credibility is his central issue, Kobren says he only allows advertisers whose products he respects. Rogaine is a regular advertiser, as is Revivogen, about which he has had "good anecdotal response."

One indication that "The Bald Truth" has become a serious industry player is that Merck recently signed on as an endorser of the show—even though Kobren tells his listeners to buy the far-cheaper Proscar and cut the 5-milligram pills into quarters.

A bigger measure of Kobren's success are the guests he books on his show. Where doctors and researchers once avoided him, lest they face criticism for not doing enough to help bald men, major clinicians and academics now readily accept Kobren's invitations to appear.

"They see that I'm giving good information and that I'm not going away," Kobren said. "I guess they decided 'If you can't beat 'em, join 'em.' "

They come on the show not just because of his solid ratings—the show is the second-highest-rated talk show in its time slot in New York—but the growing sense that Kobren is doing good in an industry that for too long has solely been concerned with selling useless medicines, treatments and information to vulnerable bald men.

Practices discussed on his show, such as the treatment of patients by New York hair transplantation surgeon Gary Hitzig, have been picked up by the mainstream media. The newsmagazine show *20/20* recently taped a segment on Hitzig, thanks to Kobren.

More important, the show has become a vital support group for many men (dozens are repeat callers who just need that pep talk). As his reputation has grown, Kobren has often been called "the Ralph Nader of Hair," but when you listen to his show, you see that he is far more similar to Richard Simmons, the chunky wild man who trimmed down and became one of the leading cheerleaders for weight loss and fat acceptance.

"This is all I do now. It's my life," Kobren says over a grilled cheese sandwich at a diner around the corner from his Manhattan apartment. "I make a living. I enjoy what I do. I enjoy being able to touch these people. They just want compassion more than anything else. They're certainly not getting it from the scientists or the physicians."

Case in point: After taking a dozen or so calls during every show, Kobren tells his listeners that he'll stay after to take a few more calls in the control room, just so those who have been on hold can get their questions answered or their emotions calmed.

One evening, he'd answered all the questions and left. A few hours later, well into the middle of the night, a woman from Canada called him at home.

"I had told the station that it was OK to give out my number, but only if the person sounded desperate, like a jumper or something," Kobren says. "And this woman was definitely upset."

The story in short: The woman's doctor had told her there was nothing he could do about her thinning hair and suggested that she just get over it and accept it. The way she told the story, the doctor told her she was wrong to feel bad about her hair loss. Funny thing was, Kobren knew the doctor and respected his work. Rather than judge the doctor, he opted merely to comfort the caller.

"I talked to her and let her know it was OK to feel bad and that there are some treatments that can work for her," Kobren says. "That's all she wanted to hear."

And then there was the e-mail Kobren received from a woman listener the day before we met at the diner. It was, naturally, unsigned, but it was titled "Pink Elephant." Kobren says it is typical of the messages he receives.

> I don't know why I took so long to write down something about this horrific ordeal I am going through. I guess it was because I didn't want to accept what I was going through . . . I am constantly faced with this unfair reality every dreadful second of the day. . . . I am only 22 and feel robbed of my self-confidence and self-esteem. . . . This has catapulted me into a deep black abyss of self-pity, sorrow and depression. On those rare days when I muster up the courage to make it out of the apartment, I feel incredibly uncomfortable. I feel like everyone is looking at my head, that they see, they know. I walk the streets of New York feeling like a giant pink elephant.

Woman or man, young or old, one thing unites Kobren's listeners, he says: "One common goal: To end their misery."

The first step is to just clear the air. Most of Kobren's callers know the minutest details about their condition and what is causing it. In fact, sitting in on one of Kobren's broadcasts, I was surprised by how well informed his listeners are about the biochemical processes that cause baldness and the pharmacological methods of preventing it.

On other late-night talk shows that I have been on, it is far more common to hear bleary guests talk about their favorite player's batting average than it is to hear men spit out phrases like "5-alpha reductase inhibitor" and "bind to the receptor site" and know what they mean, too.

Whether they want to talk about the latest snake oil—"What do you hear about human growth hormone?" asked one recent caller—or just talk about their feelings, Kobren provides the forum.

On a recent show, Lynn from New York called to say that hair loss was "driving me crazy." She said that she is in her seventies and is losing hair on the sides. She wanted to try Rogaine, but had been told that it doesn't work on the sides.

Kobren set her straight. "Upjohn can't say that it works on the sides because they never did any FDA testing for that," he said. "But we know the product does work there. There's no reason why you shouldn't try it. It may work for you."

On another show, Jim from Glendale, California, called to express concern that his lifetime of using Vitalis, a decades-old hair-styling tonic, was causing his hair loss.

"I really don't think Vitalis is a problem," Kobren said. "Men have been using Vitalis for generations. I've never heard that it causes hair loss."

A highlight of seemingly every show is the weekly conspiracy-theorist call. Yes, there is a vocal underground of bald men who sincerely believe that drug companies and researchers are stalling on finding the cure for baldness because of everything from internal company politics to lack of concern for bald men.

Go to any website and you'll read their diatribes. When the French drug company Roussel-Uclaf's baldness drug, a topical 5-alpha reductase inhibitor code named RU 58841, tested favorably in preliminary animal studies, balding men seized on the drug as the Next Big Thing. The drug got delayed when Roussel-Uclaf was bought by another pharmaceutical company, which was then bought by *another* company. Such delays are typical of the industry today—when companies can pick only a handful of drugs that they can develop in any given year—but bald men have not seen it that way.

"They don't care if we're suffering," wrote "Cueball" in a typical posting on regrowth.com, a leading baldness information site [http://www.regrowth.com]. "They don't care if we live or die. They don't care whatever outcome befalls us. They simply do not care. They won't bring the drug to market, and they won't sell it to another company that will bring it to market. . . . Aventis [the company that now owns the rights to RU 58841] is making a conscious decision to cause innocent people to suffer. The suicides are Aventis's fault. All of it."

(One man even posted the chemical formula for the compound on a website—http://www.anagen.net/ru.htm, which is great if you speak Italian—and pleaded, "We need to find a chemist who can whip up some of this stuff.")

There are many such men who used Kobren's show as a place to vent and air their conspiracy theories.

On a recent show, Pavlo from Israel phoned in with just such a purpose. He begins his call with an update on an experimental procedure called "hair multiplication," a sibling of cloning that many bald men hold out as the holy grail.

Dr. Coen Gho, a researcher in the Netherlands, is the man behind hair multiplication—but he's holed up in his lab, ever since he gave an interview to a local paper a few years ago and suddenly found himself inundated with calls, faxes, letters and e-mails from desperate bald men.

He has released no new information on his promising experiment to grow many hairs from one donor—and, indeed, did not return calls for this book, either.

Tonight, Pavlo is frustrated that Gho has not updated the millions of men hanging on his every experiment and is convinced that Gho is withholding information, although he can't quite figure out why. The inexplicable mystery is, of course, a classic part of the perfect conspiracy theory.

"He needs to see that there is a vast market for his work and that will encourage him to work even faster," Pavlo says.

This puts Kobren in a bit of an awkward position. As a beacon of hope, Kobren can ill afford to dismiss Pavlo's rantings, knowing fully well that thousands of bald men are on the same emotional roller-coaster of promising therapies and dashed hopes.

So Kobren takes a middle tack. "I'm sure that Dr. Gho realizes the importance of his work," he says.

But Pavlo is not satisfied. "We have to go to the major media and demand that they write about this," he says. "There are certain bodies out there who don't want any solution to baldness to be found.

As evidence, Pavlo explains that he was in the clinical trials of a drug called Piliel that, he claims, was working great on him—until the company shut down the trials and withdrew the drug.

"Why would they do that?" he asks rhetorically. "This was a drug that was working!"

In a subsequent e-mail exchange I had with Pavlo, he described in detail the day he went to Haifa's Technion Institute to get his monthly dose, only to be told that the experiment had been shut down and he would no longer receive the medication that was restoring his hair. Ella Lindenbaum, who conducted the tests for Piliel, described it as a gel comprised of "nutrients and growth factors required for hair growth." Lindenbaum said Piliel had similar results as Rogaine "but without any side effects," but added vaguely that the company developing the drug "failed to bring this product to market by the allotted time."

So like RU 58841, Piliel had disappeared—lost to the uncertainties of the drug-approval process and the concern that marketing the medication would ultimately be a bad long-term investment for its maker.

"I was very furious but there was nothing to do," Pavlo wrote me. "I was told by the lab workers that there were test subjects who were more extreme than me. [They] even became violent."

Whether on Kobren's radio show or in his Internet postings, Pavlo's tone is that same mix of highly combustible emotions—desperation, anger and frustration—that Kobren has experienced himself. It's like the feeling you get when your car is smacked even though you're just sitting at a red light.

But nonetheless, on this week's show, Pavlo has set the agenda. Caller after caller wants to "get back to what Pavlo was talking about," yet Kobren never loses control of his message.

"I really want to hear more about the Piliel that Pavlo was talking about," says Jim from Los Angeles. "Why isn't the drug available?"

Again, another opportunity for Kobren to show bald men that he is one of them—but yet still has enough hope in the treatments that *are* available that he is not ready to declare that the drug companies hired the second gunman on the grassy knoll.

"In some cases, it's someone in the corporate office deciding, sometimes on nothing more than a whim, that the product is not worth marketing," Kobren says, trying to strike a tone of moderation.

"Well, I must say," Jim concludes, "it does sound like there's a conspiracy going on."

A few days later, when Kobren and I meet at the diner, he explains that he empathizes with callers like Pavlo. "These are desperate people who need a scapegoat. They don't want to wait another two years."

And then he looks over at the guy sitting at the table next to us and can't believe what he's seeing. Here he is, talking about the future of curing baldness, how there's hope on the horizon, and sitting not three feet away from him is a guy with a toupee so bad that it looks as though he's wearing ear-to-ear carpeting.

"It's atrocious," Kobren says. "But he's gotten so used to it that to him, it looks fine. If he'd call my show, I'd tell him that he has to thin out the front a bit. Let's see a little scalp so it's natural-looking. This guy is in his sixties and he wants to walk around with the hairline of a twelve-year-old boy."

It's moments like these when I realize that what really drives Kobren is not merely that he sees there's a market for a hair loss therapist, but that he has a genuine passion to right the wrongs of a largely unregulated industry—the male vanity industry—filled with empty promises and shysters in lab coats.

One frequent target is Gary Hitzig, with whom Kobren got into a legal battle when he criticized the doctor on the air. (Hitzig claimed that the criticism was libelous but ultimately withdrew his complaint. Kobren stands firm in his view of Hitzig's practice.) Hitzig is not Kobren's only target, but he is a symbol of an industry that would not exist were it not for the vulnerable male ego. Thanks to competition in the hair transplant field, doctors who should limit their contact with patients simply to medical treatment are also forced to become marketers.

"A lot of their practices are just mills," Kobren complains. "And the doctors are just businessmen. My favorite was the doctor who did Nicholas Cage's transplant. He said in an interview with me that 'Cage owes me his Oscar!' That's the biggest load of crap. That was the worst hair transplant I've ever seen! Yet he markets his bad work as good work."

Of all the hair transplant surgeons in the business, Kobren takes ads only from the New Hair Institute, one of the most reputable transplant outfits. Again, credibility is Kobren's only calling card, for without it, he's just another snake-oil salesman trying to hawk a book. He's comfortable with the New Hair Institute because it doesn't recommend transplants too early; if a patient still has significant amounts of hair, the institute's medical director, Robert Bernstein, puts him on Propecia rather than initiating an expensive—and sometimes never-ending—cycle of transplants.

"I could've hooked up with the Bosley Medical Group [a nationwide hair transplant practice]," Kobren says. "They want to advertise, but Larry Lee Bosley has had his license suspended in more than a dozen states. I can't be associated with that."

The waitress comes over to refill our water glasses. She's an attractive blonde with a smile that deflects right off my wedding ring and into the single Kobren's eyes, but he just stares at her. When she walks away, I ask him what he saw.

"She has the beginnings of female pattern baldness," he says. "It's unmistakable, but I'll bet she doesn't even know it."

But, he quickly adds, ever the optimist, "By the time she notices it, there'll be plenty of treatments available. There really is hope now."

*Chapter 9*

—

# HEROISM UNDER FIRE:
# ON THE FRONT LINES FOR
# A CURE FOR BALDNESS

"Ugly is a field without grass, a plant without leaves, or a head without hair."

—OVID (43 B.C.–17 A.D.), Roman poet

D r. Coen Gho's first mistake was giving that interview.
This was back in April 1998, when Gho, a hair transplant specialist and hair biology researcher in the Netherlands, consented to be interviewed by the reputable paper *De Gelderlander* about his preliminary research in something he called "hair multiplication."

Gho's work involved a form of "cloning" premature hair-stem cells that would then each give birth to dozens of more cells to be injected (not transplanted, mind you) into the scalp. It would eliminate the need for harvesting strips of hair from the back of a man's head as in the typical hair transplant, as well as the need to crudely punch holes in the recipient sites to create new follicle sites.

The injected stem cells would form the new follicles themselves.

"In principle," the paper stated (and it's a little rough here because I'm translating from the original Dutch), "it is possible to 'grow' an infinite amount of hair follicles out of a single hair. . . . Gho says that his technique will be cheaper and more 'patient friendly' than hair transplantation."

The paper said that Gho would be treating patients "within the year." That was almost two years ago [http://www.hairsite.com/gho/drgho.htm].

So what happened? Le deluge.

Bald men are very clear about what they want: They want a cure for baldness and they want it now. So, researchers who have had even the most preliminary reports published in the most obscure scientific journals suddenly find their lives and their research turned upside down by the avalanche of interest and the level of impatience of the most vocal bald men.

When Dr. Ronald Crystal, the director of the Institute for Human Genetics at Weill Medical College of Cornell University in New York City [http://physiology.med.cornell.edu/faculty/crystal.html], demonstrated that he could stimulate the growth of hair in mice using a controversial gene-therapy procedure, he found himself on the receiving end of computer-clogging amounts of e-mail from desperate bald men begging to be included in clinical trials that would not exist for years—if they would ever exist at all.

When Dr. Angela Christiano, a genetics researcher at Columbia University, made key discoveries that could lead to the identification of the genes that cause baldness, people from all over the world started sending her batches of their own hair, dated and labeled, every month. One bald man kept leaving voice-mail messages and sending e-mails to Christiano claiming that he was a doctor who wanted to work with her. "I knew he wasn't a doctor because he spelled medical words wrong, but I called him back anyway and it turned out he was just someone who wanted to volunteer."

Just returning phone calls has kept Christiano busy—and the call volume increases whenever her name is attached to any new paper [http://cpmcnet.columbia.edu/dept/derm/labs/christiano].

When Colin Jahoda wrote a "brief communication" in the journal *Nature* last year describing his successful implantation of some of his own hair cells into his wife's forearm (which then grew hair!), he found that if he answered the volumes of mail and interview requests that he received, he could not do his work at all.

One colleague said that Jahoda has become "a total recluse now" rather than deal with the outside pressures.

Dr. Gho has largely joined those ranks as well after releasing even the most preliminary information about his research. That one article in *De Gelderlander* has kept the talk going in Internet chat rooms for more than two years.

"I contacted the clinic this month but could not get past the front desk," one bald man wrote in an Internet posting, implying that he should have been connected to Gho immediately. "The girl at the front desk said the phone was ringing all day with people asking about the process. . . . She would not let me talk with Dr. Gho."

Sympathetic? No way! The posting gave out Gho's phone number to anyone who wanted it. Many more people used it, further inundating Gho's office.

That posting was followed by one from a guy who claimed to have "spoken to Gho several times [and] heard from him that this treatment will be commercially available within one year."

But, the writer admitted, that was probably optimistic. "I don't know if I can trust this because he told the newspaper *De Gelderlander* that it will be commercially available within eight months and we know this statement didn't come true. . . . If (and this is a huge if) Gho's work is as successful as he says, anyone who will have even one percent from this research will be richer than Bill Gates."

As so often happens when information is scarce, conspiracy theories began to spring up, fueled by quick dissemination via the Internet.

"I found out that someone who visited the clinic said that Gho can clone five hairs to every one hair, then clone five more hairs to each of those hairs," wrote another man, whose vague "information" only gave rise to further excited postings and, eventually, dashed hopes. "The result is a 30-times increase of the donor area, and the hairs are cycling normally. Gho plans to teach selected doctors in 8–12 months."

Finally, Gho himself had to step in, posting a plea on the Internet for some peace and quiet. Watch how his tone becomes increasingly agitated.

"Dear interested people," he began. "Referring to all the comments, questions and phone calls I received every day about the multiplication of hairs, I hereby will give *my* comment on the new procedure we call 'Hair Multiplication.' Yes, we discovered a new method . . . but at this moment we are still in the experimental phase and want to do more research to improve the method and hairs don't grow overnight, you know?!?! We hope to have a final and practical protocol, which can be used by other physicians within a few years."

*A few years,* many bald men groaned in unison. No wonder Gho was forced to shift to uppercase letters for the rest of his posting, just so his readers would know he was serious.

"SO, I URGE YOU NOT TO CONTACT US THIS YEAR, BE-CAUSE WE PREFER TO DO THE RESEARCH STUDIES IN AN NON-STRESSFULL [sic] AND QUIET ENVIRONMENT. IT IS ALL FOR THE BEST INTEREST, BECAUSE IN THIS WAY WE CAN IMPROVE THE METHOD AS SOON AS POSSIBLE. I WILL KEEP YOU INFORMED ABOUT THE METHOD AND RESULTS. Greetings from a sunny Netherlands, Coen Gho, M.D."

That was in July 1999. Gho has not been heard from since. If that isn't bad enough, suddenly his time frame is now "within a few years"? Phrases like that are a corkscrew to the hearts of bald men.

The pressure doesn't come only from bald men, of course. After Jahoda's results—"Trans-gender Induction of Hair Follicles"—were published in *Nature,* doctors all over the world were interested. Indeed, if dermal sheath cells from one person could be successfully implanted in another without rejection, perhaps someday you'll be able to get a hair transplant from anonymous donors with geneti-cally perfect hair—any color, texture or style you like.

So in addition to bald men begging to participate in the experi-ments, doctors also besieged Jahoda. "The attitude is, if someone [read "he"] doesn't repeat this experiment, it will go down as the 'cold fusion' of hair," said George Cotsarelis, director of the Hair and Scalp Clinic at the University of Pennsylvania.

The implication is clear: Jahoda is under big-time pressure to perform. This is not how the best work—from science to art to books on baldness—is done.

Dr. Michael Holick experienced his own boomlet after publishing an esoteric paper dealing with hair cycle stimulation with parathyroid hormone-related peptide, so he knows what Gho is going through.

"I'm all over the Internet and I get e-mails from all over the place," Holick said. "That's life, but it won't change the way I do my work. I'm very interested in making sure we do excellent science. So I'm very cautious about what I do and how I do it. But bald men can be so psychologically overwhelmed that they . . ." He didn't finish the thought.

Yet despite the desperation, the future is so bright for bald men that they might want to consider picking out a barber. A veritable arsenal of assaults on male pattern baldness is in the works—from Gho's hair cloning to a new, more powerful 5-alpha reductase drug from Glaxo Wellcome to Holick's work with parathyroid-related hormones to the discovery of the genes that cause baldness itself.

On the front lines are a bunch of remarkably talented researchers and scientists who are as committed to curing baldness as their oncological colleagues are to curing cancer.

This is often a difficult thing to accept. We tend to expect scientists to constantly be at work on the most important lifesaving medication or be designing the most vital research. When honoring scientists, the awards tend to go to the people who unleash the power of the atom or uncode the human genome, not to the guy at 3M whose revolutionary research into adhesive bonding led to the invention of Post-it Notes, which, arguably, improve our lives more tangibly.

But that hasn't stopped people like genetic scientist Angela Christiano from doing their work. In Christiano's case, her interest in baldness is personal. A few years ago, overcome with the stress of a new job, turning thirty and a pending divorce, Christiano came down with alopecia areata and started losing her abundant locks in large tufts.

"I wouldn't have gotten into this were it not for my alopecia," Christiano admits. "I worked on serious skin diseases and I was one of those researchers who felt that you had to be working on something very serious to be making a difference."

It was only after she got involved in the research that she realized that the work *was* serious. "All the information about curing genetic diseases of the skin using stem cells lies in the hair follicle, so the research we're doing is elegant biology. In doing [it], we're going to learn about fundamental biological pathways and answer some profound scientific questions."

On the door of Christiano's office is a telling cartoon showing four bald doctors sitting at a dais and one at a podium. "The bad news is that after 13 years of working round-the-clock, we have discovered nothing new about cancer," the bald speaker says. "The good news is that we finally managed to isolate the gene that causes baldness."

Christiano sees the cartoon as a symbol of our love-hate relationship with the science of the supposedly trivial. The same people who make fun of the doctors who devote their lives to studying baldness someday turn forty and ask, "Why haven't you cured baldness yet?"

Christiano runs a lab of ten postdocs, students and dermatology residents. While her students run the full gamut from the standard-issue, central-casting geeks to the quiet, bookish, librarian types, Christiano is not the lab-coat-wearing sort, preferring black sweaters, black jeans and bright red nail polish.

Thanks to steroid shots in her scalp, her alopecia areata is in remission—and thanks to that remission, Christiano can affect the look she likes: a wild, Cassandra-like hairdo, the smoldering nails and the downtown-chic wardrobe.

To say that Christiano doesn't fit the mold of a geneticist is to say that Sarah Jessica Parker does not seem like a housewife. While her lab is as typical as they come—bottles labeled "70% EtOH" and "10M NaOH" fill the shelves, there are signs reading "Radioactive Material Work Area," and the place has that acid smell common in research facilities—Christiano is a bundle of energy and enthusiasm that can't be tied up in a neat bun behind horn-rimmed glasses.

"I'm happy I don't fit the mold," she says. "For a long time, people would say, 'You look like a hairdresser, not a scientist.' People didn't always take me seriously. Women doctors would pull me aside at meetings and advise me to tone it down. And I tried to look like a frump for a while, but now that we're producing solid results, I feel more free to look the way I want."

Christiano's results comprise some of the most important discoveries in the field since James Hamilton discovered the connection between hormones and baldness. Her research has helped to uncover two of the many genes that are involved in hair growth and hair loss.

To study any complex genetic condition such as male pattern baldness, researchers need to examine large numbers of siblings who are affected. Christiano began her research in Pakistan, where there had been reports of several isolated families in which several children had been born with hair that failed to regrow after it was shed for the first time, about three months after birth.

Using a technique known as linkage, which is sort of like playing a slot machine but with hundreds of thousands of numbers on dozens of wheels, Christiano and her team isolated the genes that cause the condition to an area on chromosome 8, but could not be more specific because the Human Genome Project had not yet identified all the genes on that chromosome.

Stymied, Christiano was looking for inspiration and found it in a surprising place: a lecture about sunburn. At the lecture, a scientist was talking about the hairless mouse, a genetic mutant that is used in many dermatological experiments because it grows no hair after shedding its first coat.

*It grew no hair after shedding its first coat!* Just like her Pakistani subjects.

Christiano then matched the Pakistani "hairless" gene to the gene of the hairless mouse and was able to pinpoint the mutation that blocks the regrowth of hair in these Pakistani families. It doesn't sound like much, but figuring out which genes control the still-elusive hair growth process is the final frontier of baldness research.

Once Christiano's results hit the academic journals, she started getting leads from all over the world, including one from a researcher at Harvard who told her about a tiny town in Sicily where several children exhibited the same hair abnormality as a species known as nude mice. This time, the human gene that controls the abnormality—a permanent "five o'clock shadow" look caused by the presence of pigmentation in the hair follicle, but the absence of hair itself—was identified on chromosome 17.

Neither gene seems to be directly related to male pattern baldness, but Christiano can't be sure. "So little is known about hair growth and hair cycling that we're still trying to tell the story of baldness without an alphabet," she says. "Finding these two genes are just two letters of that alphabet. Someday, we may be surprised and find that these genes actually do have some involvement in male pattern baldness."

The search for more letters of that alphabet sent Christiano to a hardscrabble region of Latin America last summer (there are better places for researchers to spend their summers, like at conferences in cushy places like Tuscany), where she met a family with some members suffering from hypertrichosis, better known as wolfmanism. Christiano's subjects were growing scalp hair all over their bodies.

In this case, the problem wasn't finding the genetic mutation that blocked hair growth, it was finding the genetic mutation that caused the follicles on the body to grow scalplike hair by mistake. The condition may relate to male pattern baldness because fetuses typically grow hair in the wolfman pattern. But a couple of months before birth, all the hair except scalp hair is shed. Perhaps male pattern baldness is just a continuation of that process.

In a year or so, Christiano believes, her team will isolate the gene that's causing the excessive hair growth—and in doing so provide another letter to mankind's slowly developing alphabet.

Rather than search willy-nilly for random letters, Ronald Crystal, who works in the cutting-edge world of gene therapy, would rather invent his own language.

Surrounded by $9 million in brand-new, state-of-the-art equipment and ensconced in the sleek offices and clean labs of the Arthur and Rochelle Belfer Gene Therapy Core Center at Weill Medical College of Cornell University in New York, Crystal is less interested in what causes diseases than he is with finding ways to cajole cells into being healthy again.

This is the state of the art in medicine right now—and Crystal's surroundings demonstrate that. His Gene Therapy Core Center is on a prime, high floor of the hospital. Where other researchers muddle along in dingy, windowless labs, Crystal's office suite has sweeping views of the East River, blond-wood desks, sleek phones and those fancy halogen desk lamps that you see in the offices of dot.com start-ups before they are forced to liquidate.

The difference between a normal lab and Crystal's center is the difference between the Russian space program and NASA. From the moment you enter, you are surrounded by technology. A digital sign in the entryway reads out the time and flashes an update, "Status OK," an indication that the incubators and refrigerators holding millions of viruses, bacteria and gene strands are running smoothly and that the entire facility doesn't have to go to DEFCON 4.

If the status were not, in fact, OK—in other words, if the temperature of those million-dollar refrigerators were to dip or rise outside the narrow parameters—the computers will automatically page the safety officer on call. If the page isn't answered, the computer will immediately call the employee at home and then move to the next person on the list until someone arrives and sets the world right again.

In the lab, young technicians and postdocs do the dirty work of gene therapy, using enzymes as molecular scissors to cut long strands of genes at precisely the right place. One technician Crystal introduces me to is filling test tubes from a beaker containing genes that may one day help induce the growth of blood vessels in the heart. For all I know, she could be filling test tubes with colored sugar solution that she'll freeze for an afternoon treat. The gene she is working on is 1,300 base-pairs long.

In an adjacent room, Crystal's technicians make viruses and then incubate them in flat flasks until needed. In such rooms, which cost $450,000 to build, the air is replaced every three minutes to avoid contamination.

The purpose of the tour is obvious, to let a visitor know that this is the future—of heart disease, cancer, even baldness. Someday, Crystal's technicians will use their enzyme scissors to cut segments of healthy genes and then inject them into a virus that will carry them to the unhealthy cells, where they are needed.

In short, damaged cells are "infected" with these disarmed cold viruses. The viruses, while unable to reproduce and take over the cell like normal viruses, are still adept at carrying genetic material—in this case, the genes that will cure whatever genetic mutation is causing your disease—into the nucleus.

That's what viruses do, after all, and that's what makes them such effective Trojan horses for gene therapy.

With baldness, Crystal and his team first determined that an already identified gene known as "sonic hedgehog" played a role in the development of embryonic hair follicles. Because the sonic hedgehog gene is involved in the growth of hair in adult mice, Crystal theorized that tricking mouse cells to overexpress sonic hedgehog would accelerate the heretofore widely misunderstood hair growth cycle.

It may sound simple, but ten years ago, the idea of putting genetic material inside a cold virus, which would then carry that genetic material into the cell nucleus, which would then incorporate it into its own genetic makeup—well, that was just science fiction.

In fact, even today, it's still a little bizarre.

"I look at a process like this," Crystal says. "Say your life depends—absolutely depends—on you delivering a letter to a Mr. Jones at the World Trade Center, but you get there and there's no directory for the World Trade Center and I won't tell you where Mr. Jones is. What would you do? You'd get as many friends as you could, Xerox the letter hundreds of times and fan out."

Before I have a chance to tell him that I might have tried something else, a megaphone, perhaps, Crystal continues. "But with disease, you can't just put the new information outside the cell because if the cell does anything, it protects its genetic information."

The solution was viruses. Once their natural propensity for overpowering cells was neutralized, viruses offered a great way of moving genes around within cells.

Crystal has already had initial success in using gene therapy to trick cells around the heart to grow new blood vessels. His team got involved with sonic hedgehog because, in addition to having a role in hair growth, the gene may also play some role in the development of skin cancer.

Crystal's team injected the sonic hedgehog–bearing virus into the mice and thought they saw follicular growth. But they couldn't be sure. After all, how do you show the acceleration of hair growth in a black mouse?

This wasn't such a small problem. Crystal surmised that the hair was growing, but he couldn't really see it. And then he had one of those "Eureka!" moments that turn science into poetry. He rounded a corner one day and checked out a bottle blonde whose dark roots were beginning to poke through. *Her dark roots were beginning to poke through!*

Crystal's next stop was to the drugstore to buy a bottle of blond hair dye for his black mice. He'd turn his mice into peroxide blondes and the new hair would grow in black, allowing him to easily monitor the different rates of hair growth between his sonic hedgehog–loaded mice and his control group.

"I've been doing research for thirty years and this is the most creative thing I've ever done," he says. "This became the only example in the literature of a bleach-blonde mouse."

The results met Crystal's hypothesis: Sonic hedgehog did accelerate the hair growth cycle. Like Christiano and her bald Pakistanis, this became front-page news and made Crystal a target. (The mouse, by the way, is long gone. It costs twenty-five cents per mouse per day to house these heroes of science and if you've got six hundred mice, the costs mount. This particular medical hero was euthanized long ago. No tickertape parade. No pat on the back, even.)

"This was in November [1999] and I still get the e-mails every week from people who want to be part of my research," Crystal says. "Men send me pictures of their heads and beg me, 'Please, can I come in and participate in a clinical trial? I don't care whether its approved or not.' "

Yet Crystal, who is quite bald, does not share many bald men's feelings of inadequacy.

"I don't know what motivates these bald men, because my bald ness doesn't bother me at all," he says. "I respect them, of course, because baldness is as important to some bald men as heart disease is to the men with heart disease."

But just as Merck waited until it could get its prostate drug, Proscar, approved before turning to its hair-growing possibilities, Crystal refuses to pursue a cosmetic application of gene therapy until the procedure itself is more widely accepted. He believes that many people are scared of gene therapy—especially in light of a death in 1999 that was linked to gene-therapy experiments—and will be until its ethical ramifications have been fully debated. He cites in vitro fertilization as a parallel. Where it was once new—and therefore suspect—IVF is now quite common.

But just as few would accept doing in vitro fertilization to ensure, for example, sex selection of the child, society is not ready to accept the risks of gene therapy—a still-untested medical procedure—to cure baldness. It could be decades before doctors are routinely inserting hair-growing genes discovered by Christiano into virus Trojan horses revolutionized by Crystal into the scalps of bald men. And Crystal is in no rush to cure baldness, anyway.

"If I have to balance doing this for baldness or heart disease, I'm doing heart disease," he says. "It takes time for society to get used to ideas. If you can't have a kid and you decide to do IVF, that's great. But twenty years ago, that wasn't possible. It takes time for people to feel comfortable with it. The history of mankind proves that science can't be stopped, but if I'm looking for a cure for cancer, I'll be able to move ahead more easily. But if someone died using [gene therapy] for baldness, there's no way to ethically justify that."

The bigger issue, of course, is that Crystal isn't even certain he could re-create the sonic hedgehog experiment in humans. "That's one of the first things you learn in medical research," Crystal says. "Human beings are not just big mice."

*Chapter 10*

—

# THEY'RE HERE, THEY'RE BARE, GET
# USED TO IT: BALD MEN ACTING UP

"There is more felicity on the far side of baldness than young men can possibly imagine."
—LOGAN PEARSALL SMITH (1865–1946), essayist

MOREHEAD CITY, N.C.—It was just the way John Capps likes it. It was Saturday night, the climactic finale of his twenty-seventh annual Bald-Headed Men of America convention. All the top honors—including the coveted Ben Franklin Look-alike Award—had already been handed out and now eighty bald men and their spouses were on their feet, singing along with a gospel band called the Believers in a slightly altered version of the hymnal "Let It Shine."

"This li'l *head* of mine, I'm gonna let it shine," the bald men sang, their voices slightly off-key, the fluorescent light bouncing off their dynamic domes. "Let it shine, let it shine, let it shine!"

This is not the way baldheaded men are supposed to behave. To the haired world, bald men are the face of ridicule. They are not supposed to be proud of their shiny pates. They are not supposed to lead well-adjusted lives with satisfied wives and happy kids.

Bald men are not supposed to line up and submit their chrome craniums to a barrage of smooches in contests for Most Kissable Bald Head, Sexiest Bald Head or Most Distinguished Bald Head. Bald men are not supposed to be able to make fun of men *with* hair, be it natural ("How do you survive the summer with that *hair?*" I was asked repeatedly) or artificial ("I feel sorry for those guys with those dead rats on their heads. They look ridiculous").

Bald men are not supposed to have a good time.

At least, that's what most people—people with hair, that is— seem to think. Bald discrimination—or at least the open mockery of the bald—is all around us, so much so, in fact, that those of us with hair probably never notice it.

But arriving in the quaint New Bern, North Carolina, airport for a gathering of bald men, I guess I was a little bit more sensitive to noticing how bald men are thought of by my fellow hair-bearers. When I told the clerk at the Budget car rental desk that I was going to the Bald-Headed Men of America convention, she just laughed. The very notion was foreign to her; imagine that, bald men getting together—and in public, no less.

"Oh, I should send my husband to that!" she said, mocking the idea that her husband would ever be proud to be bare up there. It's a typical reaction when haired people hear about baldness in general and bald pride in specific.

You can't blame the public, what with all the negative messages they hear about the bald—what with the bald industrial complex in academia and on Madison Avenue constantly portraying bald men as depressed loners with atrophied self-images who pathetically spend nearly $2 billion a year to repair themselves with toupees (rugs), hair transplants (plugs) and hair medications (drugs) in the vain hopes of one day feeling the wind blowing through their hair again.

Scholars have certainly kept themselves busy (and burned through enough grant money to light a good-sized ivory tower for years) analyzing how the typical bald man suffers from neuroses, psychoses and even the mopsies because of a lack of hair on his head.

In study after study, nonbald people looking at random pictures of men rated the baldies as uglier, less friendly and less "good" than men with hair, who were perceived as handsome, virile and active. One study—and this is my favorite, for personal reasons—showed that the hairier a man is, the more likely people will think he has a long penis. Another study even showed that bald men are far less likely to be elected to Congress (although the study unfortunately said nothing about the penis sizes of our highest elected officials).

There are two things that we can conclude from dozens of these academic studies: 1. Grant money is too easy to come by, and 2. bald men are persecuted, discriminated against and marginalized in our society.

No matter where you look—in the Bible, the history books, the psychology textbooks or even the *TV Guide*—bald men are being run down and ridiculed. Whether it was Samson becoming weak after losing his hair, Caesar shamefully covering up his naked scalp or the Visigoths scalping their defeated foes as a final humiliation, you get the message that hair loss and low self-esteem have been linked in men's minds for a very long time. And by now, it's so much a part of American culture that nobody questions it when a bald man's low self-image forms the subtext of virtually every episode of *Seinfeld.*

So it was in such an antibald context that John Capps founded the Bald-Headed Men of America in 1972. Since 1979, the group has had its annual gathering every year in Morehead City (because more head equals less hair—get it?) [http://members.aol.com/baldusa].

Capps, now fifty-nine, is the fourth generation of men in his family to go bald, but, unlike most men, the hair loss that hit him in high school never bothered him. This was the 1950s, after all, Capps said, when men didn't know the words "depression" or "trauma."

Capps has always been proud of his visible vertex and never withdrew from social settings as many bald men do. At college, he even got elected to the student council on the slogan "Vote for Bald John!" He was elected to something every year using the same bare-bones pitch.

But after college, when Capps was up for a salesman job with a company that sold stationery items to banks, the person interviewing him didn't think a guy whose hair consisted solely of earbrows could properly woo women tellers.

"It was the first time I had ever been denied an opportunity based on how I looked," he said. "I said to myself, 'Hey, there is nothing wrong with being bald, so what we need is a positive group to say 'Skin is in!' "

Now, this was back in 1972 and skin was definitely not in. This was the era of hair, hair and more hair, when being bald was not the fashion statement it has been since Michael Jordan turned his own hair loss into the biggest thing since double-sided toupee tape. This was the 1970s! The Sexual Revolution was on—and men without hair were definitely on the losing side.

"I went bald in the late sixties when I was twenty-one," said Walker McWee, attending his seventh-straight convention. "If you had even a small bald spot, you were considered too old to date."

Back then, before he knew what he knows now, McWee did something that shames him today: He actually bought a hairpiece, his concession to the brutal capitalism of the dating market. But he threw it away after only two weeks.

"I decided, if they didn't like me for *me,* I didn't want to know them," he said with pride.

It's people like McWee whom Capps has sought out. Networking like the Chamber of Commerce director he once was, Capps printed up simple brochures and cajoled people to let him put them into those tourist-trap racks at rest stops, hotels and restaurants up and down the so-called Crystal Coast (the region, it turns out, was named a decade ago at a Chamber meeting in, of course, Capps's house).

When a reporter from the now defunct *National Observer* came to North Carolina to cover the national pig hollering contest in a neighboring town, he heard about Capps and returned a few months later to write up a story about the Bald-Headed Men. That started the media bandwagon rolling, and Capps increasingly got noticed by newspapers and magazines and found himself called upon to fill the hungry maw of the Donahue–Geraldo–Morton Downey, Jr. circuit.

The big break came in 1976, when the mayor of St. Louis invited Capps and Co. to celebrate the nation's bicentennial under the Gateway Arch, a fittingly shaped symbol.

The rest is not only history, but a great story.

"Next thing I knew, the producer of that show *Real People* called

me up and asked where the *next* Bald-Headed Men of America convention would be. Now, I didn't have a convention planned, so I said,
'It's right here in Morehead City,' and I even made the 'more
head/less hair' joke. Of course, I was making it all up. I didn't have
another convention planned. I was just winging it for this big producer. So he said, 'Great. We're going to put you on this new show
called *Real People.*' Well, at that point, we *had* to have a convention."

Now, Capps said, his group is "boasting more than thirty thousand members"—although such numbers seem to be just that, a
boast, when you're sitting in two adjacent conference rooms at the
Morehead City Hampton Inn with a mere thirty-five bald guys. But
the Bald-Headed Men of America make up for their questionable
numbers with enthusiasm and puns.

"We're the only group that grows because of a lack of growth,"
Capps is fond of saying. "We invite the media to cover the uncov-
ered at our hair-raising event. If you don't got it, flaunt it."

The media are as big a part of Capps's annual gathering as the
twenty-five or so regulars and ten newcomers who show up. Thirty-
five bald men and their families do not a revolution make—but
when the sights and sounds of them whooping it up are broadcast
across the country, they lend all the trappings of a movement.

Capps is more showman than crusader, more P. T. Barnum than
Pat Buchanan. His goal is not to establish a bald pride movement or
foment a revolution. Capps just wants to have a good time with his
friends, tell them that they're just as good, just as manly as other
men, and give them a booster shot if they're weakening.

One way of doing that is to provide TV and the print media
plenty of great photo ops of bald men carousing—even if the
carousing is just for the cameras. A good portion of the convention
is spent giving interviews and getting out the message of bald pride.
The rest is, quite frankly, just spent sitting around chewing the fat
(and, when you're in North Carolina, there's plenty of fat to chew).
In that way, perhaps, the Bald-Headed Men of America is a classic
support group; a weekend in Morehead City isn't packed with fun-
filled, action-heavy events. It's all about the company.

The weekend of bald pride begins with a preconvention, get-reacquainted dinner at a local restaurant on Thursday night. This year, Capps picked the venue perfectly; Magnolia Tree Cafe owner Ruthie King, all three hundred pounds of her, is the embodiment of the Bald-Headed Men of America's subliminal message that people must be taken for who they are, not whom society wills them to be.

"You may notice that I'm overweight, but because I'm open about who I am, I've been able to date whatever man I've wanted," she said, an inspiration to anyone anywhere who is not perfect. "I'm not vain and I don't want to be with a vain man, so no toupees or hair transplants, thank you very much."

And, she explained, she loves to go skinny-dipping with them because when she holds a bald guy to her chest, "it looks like I have three boobs."

Is that a good thing?

"That's a good thing," she said.

It's a lot better than dating a guy with a bad hair transplant, that's for sure. King recalled a recent boyfriend whose huge beach house turned her on, but whose pluggy transplants turned her off.

"We were in bed once—nothing had happened yet, if you must know—and he started futzing with one of the plugs," she recalled. "I said to myself, 'I have to get out of here right now. This beach house isn't worth it.' But these guys here, these bald guys, are good human beings with warm hearts. That means everything to me."

Here it comes, the sex thing. With so much bald pride on display—and, indeed, so much testosterone around—there's naturally plenty of boasting about the long-proclaimed but little-proven side benefits to being bald men.

"See this?" McWee said, burnishing his bald head with a piece of chamois. "This is a solar panel for a sex machine."

Baldness is, to some extent, caused by male sex hormones, so there may be some truth to these guys' claim that bald men are just plain better in the sack.

"I've never dated a bald man before and now I'll never go back," said Linda Jacobs, who accompanied baldy David Stevenson, her boyfriend of eight months. "Look at that head! Touch it, kiss it, caress it."

When I declined her invitation (much to Stevenson's relief), Jacobs said there's nothing better than lathering up her man's head, shaving it down and toweling it off. "It's fun and sensual," she said.

Fearing I'd started something I couldn't finish, I sought out Cynthia Falgiano, who had also never dated a bald man until she met Bob Frimstone (this year's Sexiest Bald Head award winner).

"I always said I'd never date a bald man," she said. "I just didn't find it attractive. Even after I met Bob and liked him, I didn't think I could do it. But meeting Bob has definitely changed my life."

There's your slogan for next year's convention: "Bald Men: Changing America's Women One Head at a Time."

Friday is media day, and a contingent of baldies hit the local talk radio station to wave the flag and pull in last-minute guests for the all-day Saturday festivities (hey, bald men never have dates on Saturday night so they'll be free, right?).

This year, Capps is too busy handling other media requests to head to the studios of 107.3 FM for the morning show with host Ben Ball ("Coastal daybreak on WTFF, the voice of Carteret County!"), so three baldies and one reporter who happens to be working on a book about baldness are dispatched to the studio to give Ball and his listeners a view of the future. Ball claims that his own baldness doesn't bother him, but he resists several invitations to come to the convention. He has a great scalp for radio, that guy.

John Capps would call him—and, indeed, *has* called him—a "baldy in training."

Like any media personality not quite ready for prime time, Ball doesn't really know what to ask the bald men other than questions like "So, this bald thing. What's the deal?"

Finally, Ball manages to lob McWee a softball about how baldness wasn't cool until Michael Jordan made it cool.

Home run: "Michael Jordan couldn't have made it cool until *we* made it cool," McWee says. "We were waiting fifteen years for the rest of the world to catch up with us."

McWee is an interesting character. Overweight, bald, asthmatic, he is hardly the stereotypical vision of an activist. But when he's not celebrating the bald, he's also a champion of the Sons of Confederate Veterans, another pride group dedicated to another misunderstood bunch of fellows [http://www.scv.org].

For McWee, both issues—bald pride, Confederate pride—are part of the same issue that Ruthie King was talking about: understanding who we are as people. McWee's flag waving (and we're talking the Confederate flag here) can get overbearing and needlessly provocative, but whether he's talking about being proud of his baldness or being proud of his ancestors who fought in the Confederate Army, all he's really saying is this is who he is. It's not perfect, but it can't be ignored either.

It's about changing perceptions. So when Ball wonders how bald men can stand in the wind without getting cold, McWee immediately corrects this misperception.

"You'd think that, wouldn't you, but when you have no hair, there's no hair to move when the wind blows," he says. "We feel the wind less than you do."

By now, Capps has set up the bald boutique, a combination registration desk and emporium where he sells novelty items such as "Bald Is Beautiful" T-shirts, special scalp razors (the secret is the handle), pate polishers and bald-man combs (sides only).

Every once in a while, Capps has to do an interview for another TV or radio station. On this particular morning, he's facing questions from a nervous rookie seemingly on her first assignment. Capps has been interviewed so many times—by the BBC, PBS, the Discovery Channel, *20/20, Nightline,* etc.—that he barely even waits for her to finish asking the question before he launches into his made-for-TV patter like a carnival barker. He knows what to say, and, more important, he knows what collection of sound bites is right for each media outlet.

"When we started twenty-seven years ago, if you were bald, they wouldn't hire you, but now, bald people are getting ahead! There are still a lot of people who fight it, who don't want us to go bald. It's a billion-dollar industry selling us combs, shampoos, hairpieces, hair transplants, hair medication, but this is a celebration of skin and who we are."

Anything else? the reporter asks nervously.

"This is a day of skin and skin is in!"

Anything else? She's not really listening to the answers, just making sure the tape is rolling. What he's saying, in essence, doesn't matter as long as she's getting it.

"You know, I don't have anything against a bald man who feels he needs to wear a toupee or get a hair transplant, I really don't. But we're offering those guys an alternative that's much cheaper: acceptance. It's all about the media, of course: All those toupee ads, they tell the whole story. They'll say, 'We'll make you look younger.' Who wants to look younger? The media is telling us we have to look younger. No, I say we should look good, but look our age. The only people who think we need to look younger are the people who are trying to sell us *products* to make us look younger."

Later, he conducts what is shamelessly billed as the Bald Man Photo Op over at the offices of his eponymous printing shop. Capps's three-building complex is located, of course, on Bald Drive, which Capps named because it's a private road, not because he paid off some local official.

"It's the only road in town that's not paved," he says. "It's bald, too!"

On Bald Drive, Capps long ago installed a three-level riser to make his annual Bald Man Photo Op quick and easy. He even has it deployed directly under the Bald Drive road sign and at the perfect angle so that even the rookie photographers can capture the bald heads, the road sign and the Morehead City water tower all in the same frame.

"OK, let's moon 'em," Capps says, instructing his fellow baldies to lean forward so that their naked heads are the dominant feature of every photo. When I aimlessly flip through the photo albums Capps keeps in the office, I see that he has staged the same photos every year for more than a decade.

The Bald-Headed Men of America is billed as a self-help group, but no one attending this three-day Baldstock needs any help dealing with their natural condition. They've long since abandoned any emotional attachment to their hair, adhering instead to a modified version of the old ACT-UP slogan: "We're here, we're bare, get used to it!"

"I'm a man of science, so I realize it's futile to try to cure something that is totally natural," says Bruce Wartham, the Ben Franklin look-alike, who is an environmental chemist and comes to the convention every year from Columbus, Ohio. Wartham is a perfect example of the kind of man John Capps wants to help. Awkward by disposition and a loner in his choice of hobbies (biking and caving), Wartham does not experience this kind of fellowship the other 363 days of the year.

His license plate reads "Bald Bat" and he certainly lives the part of an animal with a decidedly different set of active senses. He needs his fellow baldies, if only because the sitting around and talking this weekend provide the most affectionate conversations he'll have all year.

"This kind of thing is very important for a guy like Bruce," Capps says. "There is a human element to this whole thing. It's the only place he can be himself without anyone judging him—because we've all been there in one way or another." The only bald-related thing not welcome at this convention is a comb-over.

Capps tells another story of a member who suffers from cerebral palsy, which affects him much more than his baldness. His condition makes him a bit of an outcast—I even found myself avoiding asking him questions, completely due to my own stupid prejudice about people with so-called "special needs"—but Capps won't allow anyone to be marginalized at his convention.

One year, Capps called him up to the stage to lead the group in the Pledge of Allegiance. "His wife later told me that it was the first time anyone had ever called upon him to do anything," Capps says. "She said he never forgot it and it's helped draw him out."

Such moments are the centerpiece of Capps's entire weekend. Every member of the group gets up on stage at some point, if only

to be kissed on the head by the judges, receive a proclamation to sig-
nify attendance or accept an award like Best Bald-Headed Smile or
Best Fringes. Like a classic roast, the microphone is open and Capps
is the kind of generous toastmaster who doesn't care who gets credit
for the joke as long as everyone is laughing.

But unlike a classic roast, no one is on the spot here.

The convention hall is actually two Hampton Inn conference
rooms—the Pamlico Room and the Bogue Room—without the di-
vider that usually separates them. In advance, Capps has strung up
plastic flags of the world, like you'd see at the opening of an ice
cream parlor, to lend an international feel.

There's no set agenda, except that everyone gets mentioned at
some point. Whenever Capps is stuck for material, he calls upon the
Believers to sing another song ("Jesus built a bridge to heaven, the
very best he could/With only three nails and two pieces of wood!"
are the implausible lyrics of one song).

It is not lost on this crowd that Harry, the lead singer, is almost totally bald.

"I believe you have some wavy hair still up there, Harry," Capps
says as the group leaves the stage. "Well, it's waving good-bye,
buddy."

(McWee, watching the scene, jokes, "Next year, instead of the
Believers, John should just play the Doors' 'People Are Strange.'
That should be our theme song. We're a strange group of guys.")

Next up, longtime member Frank Baumet offers the "Room 101
Report," an inside joke at every convention for the last five years,
ever since one member and his wife conceived their first child while
staying in the fabled room. Since that night, any time any of these
baldies wants to mention sex, all he has to do is say "Room 101."

Of course, none of the jokes means anything to the outsider—
"Hey, Frank, you got a red car, right?"—but you spend three hours
laughing anyway.

Capps then calls upon Jim Dyer of Wake Forest, North Carolina,
to reiterate the group's mission statement. "Some of you think our
only purpose is to provide bald heads for [judge] Judy Wessel to

kiss, but we do have a more important purpose," Dyer says before embarking on a long pause meant to indicate that for the life of him, he doesn't know or care what that "important" purpose is.

Finally, he turns around to read the text off one of Capps's posters. "Oh, yeah, our purpose is that we are a 'self-help, service club founded in 1972 dedicated to "Bald Is Beautiful." ' "

But later, Dyer, a minister, leads his slick-topped congregation in a prayer of thanks to God for "making us in Your image"—an interesting concept in a world where the Lord and His Son are unfailingly depicted as possessors of truly heavenly heads of hair.

And the climax of the convention is, of course, the judging, when "head" judge Wessel gets to do her thing, loading up her lips with bright red lipstick and kissing every scalp in sight.

"I love to kiss bald heads," Wessel says. None of the men removes the residue of the kiss for hours, preferring to wear it as a badge of honor.

It's telling in this Internet age that the Bald Poobah of the Bald-Headed Men doesn't even maintain a website. While more and more Americans seek out like-minded souls on the World Wide Web—and, indeed, there are bald pride websites such as balditude.com and powerbalding.com—Capps is striking a blow against digital America, preferring the glare bouncing off his conventioneers' heads to the glow of virtual reality. His "chat room" is the Pamlico Room at Morehead City's Hampton Inn, all dolled up with bald pride posters, not some digitized home page with downloadable photos of other people having fun. Maybe he doesn't have thirty thousand members, but he has a following far more vast than even the best advocacy websites, which, no matter how credible or how professional they look, always plant in my head the image of an angry loner banging out rants that are read by him alone.

To Capps, no Internet site—no herky-jerky streaming video—is as satisfying as a handshake or the feeling of a big, wet kiss being planted on a smooth, bald head.

It feels like a movement.

# Acknowledgments

The contents of this book would have been dramatically diminished were it not for the help of many people who lent me aid, comfort and pizza during the writing. First, my editors at the *New York Post* deserve special commendation for indulging me during the writing of this book and not grumbling when my bald men suddenly started making regular appearances in my weekly column. I'd like to offer my thanks to the entire staff at the New York Academy of Medicine, whose library is open, free to the public, every day. I spent many weeks sitting there reading medical journals and found the library staff attentive, helpful and committed. I would also like to thank Robert Tenuta, who minds the American Medical Association's historical frauds collection, where I did much of the research on the snake-oil era. While I think it is appalling that the AMA charges researchers to look through its collection, I remain thankful to Tenuta for helping me wade through it. I'd also like to single out John Capps, the president and founder of the Bald-Headed Men of America, for doing more than merely inviting me to Morehead City, North Carolina, for the group's annual convention. Capps made me feel welcome—even though I, in fact, have hair.

I am indebted also to the many medical professionals who helped me make sure that what I wrote actually conformed to what I thought I understood from our discussions. I'd like to offer special thanks to Dr. Angela Christiano at Columbia University; Rogaine legend "Mac" Corum; Norman Orentreich, the father of the hair transplant; Elliot Nonas, the most honest man in toupees today;

Robert Bernstein of the New Hair Institute; and Daniel Moerman of the University of Michigan, who, when I asked for some information about Rogaine, sent me an entire binder of scientific reports from a 1988 symposium at Upjohn's Kalamazoo headquarters. The group photo of the symposium participants—what hair!—kept me happy for days.

Special thanks are due to my editor at Random House, Jon Karp, who did a big favor to a journalist "in between jobs," and my agent, Simon Lipskar, who got me paid for it.

I'd also like to thank my talented colleagues who talked me through the writing: Lawrence Goodman, Stephanie Dolgoff, Andrew Corsello, Kurt Hirsch and Carol Hamburger (for the pizza), George Plimpton and David Shenk.

# Web Resources Directory

ABC News—Hugh Downs bio
[http://www.abcnews.go.com/onair/2020/downs_hugh_bio.html]
Bald Headed Men of America
[http://members.aol.com/baldusa]
The Bald Truth
[http://www.thebaldtruth.com]
The Bald Truth radio show
[http://www.thebaldtruth.org/html/radio_shows.htm]
Biblical Studies Foundation
[http://www.bible.org]
Thomas F. Cash, Ph.D., website
[http://www.body-images.com/main.html]
Center for Drug Evaluation and Research's Gallery of Nostrums
[http://www.fda.gov/cder/about/history/gallery/gallery1.htm]
Dr. Angela Christiano website
[http://cpmcnet.columbia.edu/dept/derm/labs/christiano]
Dr. Coen Gho's Hair Multiplication Procedure
[http://www.hairsite.com/gho/drgho.htm]
Dr. Ronald G. Crystal website
[http://physiology.med.cornell.edu/faculty/crystal.html]
DermMatch
[http://www.dermatch.com]
The Eagles' Gallery
[http://www.eaglesmusic.com/gallery/bwcover.html]
The Hair Advocates Network
[http://www.hairadvocates.com/nhscale.html]

Hair Club for Men
[http://www.hairclub.com]
Hairsite.com RU 58841 topic
[http://www.hairsite.com/disc177_toc.htm]
Hitzig & Schwinning Medical Group
[http://www.877hairusa.com]
Merck
[http://www.merck.com]
National Alopecia Areata Foundation
[http://www.alopeciaareata.com]
New Hair Institute
[http://www.800newhair.com]
Norwood & Lehr Hair Transplant Clinic
[http://www.hairclinic.com]
Orentreich Medical Group
[http://www.orentreich.com]
Penguin Place
[http://www.penguin-place.com]
The Penthouse for Hair Recovery
[http://www.penthousehair.com]
Pharmacia & Upjohn
[http://www.pnu.com]
Regrowth.com
[http://www.regrowth.com]
Revivogen website
[http://www.revivogen.com]
Ronco.com
[http://www.ronco.com]
RU 58841 chemical formula website
[http://www.anagen.net/ru.htm]
Sons of Confederate Veterans
[http://www.scv.org]
Spencer Forrest's Solutions for Hair Loss
[http://www.toppik.com]
Wolfman Jack Photo Gallery
[http://www.wolfmanjack.org/picgal.htm]

# About the Author

Gersh Kuntzman has been a reporter for the *New York Post* since 1993, first covering the entertainment industry and later writing news features. Since 1995, he has been a columnist for the paper. His weekly column, "Metro-Gnome," provides a witty and wry slice-of-life take on New York City. Several of his features have won awards, and a series of articles on the annual hot dog eating contest at Coney Island was turned into an award-winning film, *Red, White and Yellow*. His freelance writing has appeared in *Cosmopolitan, Glamour, The New York Observer, George, Salon, New York* magazine and *Modern Humorist. Hair! Mankind's Historic Quest to End Baldness* is his first book. He is not bald. He apologizes.

## About AtRandom.com Books

AtRandom.com books are original publications that make their first public appearance in the world as e-books, followed by a trade paperback edition. AtRandom.com books are timely and topical. They exploit new technologies, such as hyperlinks, multimedia enhancements, and sophisticated search functions. Most of all, they are consumer-powered, providing readers with choices about their reading experience.

AtRandom.com books are aimed at highly defined communities of motivated readers who want immediate access to substantive and artful writing on the various subjects that fascinate them.

Our list features literary journalism; fiction; investigative reporting; cultural criticism; short biographies of entertainers, athletes, moguls, and thinkers; examinations of technology and society; and practical advice. Whether written in a spirit of play or rigorous critique, these books possess a vitality and daring that new ways of publishing can aptly serve.

For information about AtRandom.com Books and to sign up for our e-newsletters, visit www.atrandom.com.